GLAUCOMA

GLAUCOMA

Pierre Blondeau, M.D.

Paul Harasymowycz, M.D.

With contributions by Patrick Hamel, M.D. to Chapter 2

In collaboration with Frédérique David

Preface by Andrew C.S. Crichton

AP Annika Parance Publishing

AP Annika Parance Publishing
1043 Marie-Anne Street East
Montreal, Quebec H2J 2B5
514-658-7217
apediteur.com

English translation: Debby Dubrofsky
Book and cover design: Francis Desrosiers in collaboration with Scalpel Design
Cover photograph: iStockphoto/Medlar

Photographs and illustrations courtesy of Alcon Canada Inc. (pages 107), Allergan Inc. (pages 31, 33, 35, 45, 51, 81 [bottom], 83 [bottom], 99, 101 and 105), Pierre Blondeau, M.D. (pages 75, 77, 79, 81 [top], 83 [top] and 109) and Glaukos Corporation (page 113)

Bibliothèque et Archives nationales du Québec and Library and Archives Canada cataloguing in publication

Blondeau, Pierre, 1950-
    [Glaucome. English]
    Glaucoma
    (Understand the disease and its treatment)
    Translation of : Glaucome.
    ISBN 978-2-923830-20-9

    1. Glaucoma - Popular works. I. Harasymowycz, Paul, 1971-   . II. Title. III. Title : Glaucome. English. IV. Series : Understand the disease and its treatment.

RE871.B5613 2014   617.7'41   C2013-942167-X

Legal deposit - Bibliothèque et Archives nationales du Québec, 2014
Legal deposit - Library and Archives Canada, 2014

Printed in Canada

Glaucoma is a disease that leads to gradual loss of sight without notice-able symptoms in the beginning. Many people who have glaucoma do not understand the importance of treating the disease. This book, I hope, will give them a better understanding of glaucoma and help them through the different stages of treatment. I would like to thank the editorial and publishing team for their indefatigable assistance. My thanks as well to my wife, Claire, for her unending support.

Pierre Blondeau, M.D.

I dedicate this book to my parents and grandparents, who sacri-ficed everything to immigrate to Canada so their children could have the best possible education. I also want to thank the many patients, teachers, colleagues and students with whom I continue to learn daily about our extraordinary sense of sight and who give me the passion and energy to continue teaching and researching the best methods for the detection and treatment of glaucoma. I especially want to thank my wife Nataliya, and my children Emilia, Sophia and Julian, with whom I am fortunate to continue this excit-ing journey.

Paul Harasymowycz, M.D.

The publisher would like to thank Josée Blondeau, Psychologist, and Julie-Andrée Marinier, Optometrist and Low Vision Specialist at the Institut Nazareth et Louis-Braille in Montreal, for their invalu-able advice concerning Chapter 6.

CONTENTS

CHAPTER 2
FORMS AND SYMPTOMS   **41**

CHAPTER 3

RISK FACTORS 57

CHAPTER 4

DIAGNOSIS 69

CHAPTER 6
LIVING WITH GLAUCOMA 117

LIST OF BOXES

THE AUTHORS

Pierre Blondeau, M.D.
Dr. Pierre Blondeau is a full clinical professor at the University of Sherbrooke. He received his training in glaucoma at the University of Iowa and has been practicing and teaching at the Sherbrooke university health centre (CHUS) since then. He has also served as academic director and head of ophthalmology at CHUS.

In addition to acting as a reviewer for a number of professional journals, Dr. Blondeau has published more than 60 research studies and given more than 160 presentations—provincially, nationally and internationally. The excellence of his research and his commitment to teaching have earned him numerous awards.

Dr. Blondeau has been dedicated to educating people with glaucoma for many years. Aware of the disastrous consequences when those with glaucoma fail to treat their disease out of ignorance, Dr. Blondeau established information sessions for patients that have been attended by more than 1,500 participants. He also produced a teaching DVD (*Vivre avec le glaucome*) for people with glaucoma to complement the information sessions. This book is a continuation of his educational mission.

Paul Harasymowycz, M.D.

Dr. Paul Harasymowycz heads the glaucoma research unit at the University of Montreal and has served as clinician and researcher at the Maisonneuve-Rosemont Hospital and the Guy-Bernier Research Centre since 2011. He is medical director of the Bellevue ophthalmology clinics and the Montreal Glaucoma Institute. He is also medical director of the Quebec Glaucoma Foundation, an organization dedicated to promoting glaucoma research in Quebec, increasing public awareness of the disease and educating people who suffer from the illness.

Dr. Harasymowycz's research focuses on glaucoma screening, new diagnostic technologies and new surgical treatments for glaucoma and cataracts. He has a passion for teaching students, residents and glaucoma fellows and is often invited to present and teach surgical techniques at national and international conferences. He is a member of the Glaucoma Committee of the American Society of Cataract and Refractive Surgery (ASCRS) and sits on the board of directors of the Association des Médecins Ophtalmologistes du Québec (Quebec's association of ophthalmologists). He has published over fifty articles in peer-reviewed medical journals as well as book chapters on glaucoma.

SPECIAL CONTRIBUTOR TO CHAPTER 2, *GLAUCOMA IN CHILDREN*

Patrick Hamel, M.D.

A pediatric ophthalmologist, Dr. Patrick Hamel is head of the ophthalmology department at Sainte-Justine Hospital and also directs the University of Montreal's ophthalmology residency program. After a postdoctoral fellowship in pediatric ophthalmology at the University of Toronto and then a subspecialization in glaucoma, he took charge of the pediatric glaucoma clinic at the University of Montreal.

Dr. Hamel is a frequent conference lecturer on the subject of childhood glaucoma. He also teaches at a number of universities. He is a member of the Childhood Glaucoma Research Network (CGRN). The genetics of childhood glaucoma is his main focus of interest.

PREFACE

Any book on the subject of glaucoma meant to give patients a better understanding of the condition would be a valuable contribution to the management of this difficult disease. Glaucoma is an asymptomatic condition until it is too late. As a result, it is essential for patients to comprehend the disease if they are to comply with treatments that can be expensive, accompanied by side effects and, in rare cases, associated with disastrous complications. For the patient to feel comfortable and adhere to the treatment plan, it is crucial that the individual and the family understand what the disease is and why it must be treated.

To this end, Dr. Pierre Blondeau and Dr. Paul Harasymowycz have done a wonderful job in putting together a book intended to explain the condition to patients and to answer many of the frequently asked questions. The layout and flow of the book are to be commended, with its clear articulation of common questions followed by brief, easily understood answers. The chapters transition very well with some of the major points highlighted by case histories—a marvellous technique for enhancing patient understanding of the condition. I will most certainly use this patient education book routinely in my practice.

Drs. Blondeau and Harasymowycz have a long history of patient advocacy, highlighted by the extensive patient education programs offered in Sherbrooke by Dr. Blondeau. I am delighted that these long-standing efforts have now been put into a format that will reach a wider audience.

Andrew C.S. Crichton, M.D., F.R.C.S.C
Clinical Professor of Surgery,
Division of Ophthalmology,
Faculty of Medicine, University of Calgary

25 FREQUENTLY ASKED QUESTIONS

(1) What are the forms and symptoms of glaucoma?
Excluding borderline glaucoma (glaucoma suspect) and childhood glaucoma, there are two main forms of glaucoma: open-angle glaucoma and angle-closure glaucoma. There are generally no symptoms in either of these forms of the disease. There is no pain, no loss of vision (except in the advanced stage of the disease) and the eye looks normal. Left undiagnosed, glaucoma may continue to progress for years without the patient's knowledge, causing the destruction of optic nerve fibre and an irreversible loss of sight. Symptoms appear only in case of an acute angle-closure glaucoma attack, which occurs suddenly and causes severe pain, vision loss and sometimes nausea and vomiting. An acute angle-closure glaucoma attack is an ophthalmological emergency. Fortunately, such attacks are very rare (*Chapter 2*).

(2) Is glaucoma a common disorder?

Glaucoma affects one to three percent of the population of the Western world age 40 and over. An estimated 400,000 Canadians have glaucoma. According to the World Health Organization, glaucoma is the second leading cause of blindness in the world, after cataracts.

The incidence of glaucoma increases with age, rising from two percent in people over age 40, to five percent in those over 65 and ten percent in people over 80 (*Chapter 1* and *Chapter 3*).

(3) How can I know if I have glaucoma?

As glaucoma is an asymptomatic disease, the importance of regular eye examinations by an optometrist cannot be overemphasized, especially if you are over 40 and have one or more risk factors. The Canadian Ophthalmological Society recommends that anyone at risk of glaucoma (with a family history of glaucoma, for example) have an eye examination at least every three years over age 40, at least every two years over age 50 and at least every year over age 65 (*Chapter 2* and *Chapter 4*).

(4) How can I know if I am a glaucoma suspect?

As the name suggests, a glaucoma suspect is a patient who may be at risk of developing glaucoma because he or she shows signs of glaucoma or has one or more glaucoma risk factors. Only a doctor can determine if you are a glaucoma suspect (*Chapter 2*).

(5) What causes glaucoma?

The genes and mechanisms responsible for glaucoma have not all been identified. As a result, we do not yet know the exact causes of glaucoma. However, several risk factors (elevated eye pressure being the most common) whose presence promotes the onset of glaucoma have been identified (*Chapter 3*).

⑥ Is glaucoma contagious or hereditary?

Glaucoma is not caused by an infection, so there is no risk that you might catch it from someone else. However, several people in the same family may have glaucoma due to a family predisposition to the disease (*Chapter 3*).

⑦ Does glaucoma cause blindness?

Glaucoma that is not treated, no matter what the form of the disease, may end in blindness. It is only a matter of time (several years) before eyesight is lost if glaucoma is left untreated. An acute angle-closure glaucoma attack can cause loss of sight within days. Such attacks are an ophthalmological emergency and are fortunately rare (*Chapter 2*).

⑧ If I have elevated intraocular pressure, does that mean I have glaucoma?

Not all cases of glaucoma are accompanied by elevated intraocular pressure (IOP). There are people who have elevated intraocular pressure for many years yet never develop glaucoma. Conversely, there are people with normal or even low intraocular pressure who have glaucoma. In other words, intraocular pressure is not the only factor in the development of glaucoma (*Chapter 2* and *Chapter 3*).

⑨ Can glaucoma be caused by an accident or a disease?

Yes. There are secondary glaucomas that are caused by trauma to the eye. Also, some diseases, and their treatments, can cause glaucoma, mainly joint inflammation disorders that cause intraocular pressure to rise (*Chapter 2* and *Chapter 3*).

⑩ Is glaucoma caused by overuse of the eyes?

No. Glaucoma is not caused by reading for long periods of time, working at a computer, watching television or precision activities requiring intense use of the eyes (*Chapter 3*).

⑪ Can high blood pressure cause glaucoma?

No. High blood pressure can cause a slight increase in intraocular pressure, but not enough to provoke glaucoma (*Chapter 3*).

⑫ Can glaucoma be prevented?

The only type of glaucoma that can be prevented is acute angle-closure glaucoma attack. An iridotomy (microscopic hole in the iris) can be performed as a preventive measure. For all other types of glaucoma, there is no preventive therapy (*Chapter 5*).

⑬ Can glaucoma be cured?

No. At present, glaucoma cannot be cured. Even after an iridotomy (laser procedure), regular follow-up by an ophthalmologist or an optometrist is required, because angle-closure glaucoma can turn into open-angle glaucoma if elevated intraocular pressure persists. In addition, damage to the optic nerve caused by glaucoma is irreversible. However, if diagnosed and treated sufficiently early, glaucoma can be kept under good control in most cases (*Chapter 5*).

⑭ Can the progression of glaucoma be slowed?

Yes. There are very effective treatments available that can slow the progression of glaucoma. A variety of surgical procedures can be used to drain the aqueous humour from the eye and lower intraocular pressure. Trabeculectomy is the most common type of surgery. There are also a number of laser procedures that can be used in different types of glaucomas, notably iridotomy in the treatment of angle-closure glaucoma (*Chapter 5*).

⑮ Can I stop using my eye drops if I feel weak and my eyes are red?

Unless instructed otherwise, it is dangerous to stop using your eye drops for any extended length of time. When the treatment is discontinued, intraocular pressure rises and vision gradually deteriorates. You must tell your attending care team of any side effects you experience. Often there are other medical or surgical solutions for reducing intraocular pressure (*Chapter 5*).

16 How often should I see my ophthalmologist?

Anyone who has glaucoma must be followed by an ophthalmologist. Your ophthalmologist will tell you what treatment you require and how often you need to see him or her based on the type and stage of your glaucoma (*Chapter 4*).

17 If one eye is affected, will the other automatically be affected?

Most of the time, both eyes are affected, though not necessarily to the same degree. Some types of glaucoma, however, can affect only one eye, particularly angle-closure glaucoma, exfoliative glaucoma and post-traumatic glaucoma (*Chapter 2*).

18 Can glaucoma be triggered by certain drugs?

Yes. Taking certain drugs increases the risk of glaucoma. Use of cortisone can reveal or trigger open-angle glaucoma in people predisposed to it. Angle-closure glaucoma suspects (*see Question 4*) should also avoid certain drugs that can dilate the pupil and trigger an acute angle-closure glaucoma attack. Such an attack is an ophthalmological emergency and can very quickly lead to blindness. However, it is recommended that you consult your doctor before discontinuing any treatment (*Chapter 2* and *Chapter 3*).

19 Can the vision loss be corrected by eyeglasses?

No. The damage to the visual field caused by glaucoma is irreversible. No eyeglasses can compensate for the vision loss nor can it be restored by any treatment. Compliance with the treatment prescribed by your doctor is thus crucial, even when no symptoms are felt, to avoid permanent damage (*Chapter 5* and *Chapter 6*).

⃝20 Can I drive if I have glaucoma?

Yes. Most people with glaucoma can keep their driver's licence for a very long time, as their vision is not affected.

Driving only becomes difficult and dangerous in very advanced glaucoma. If the damage to the optic nerve and the visual field loss are substantial, the ophthalmologist and the licensing authority may decide that the patient is unable to drive safely and will have to give up his or her driver's licence permanently (*Chapter 6*).

⃝21 Can I wear contact lenses if I have glaucoma?

Wearing contact lenses is not a problem for most people with glaucoma. Exceptions are those who have had certain types of surgery after which the wearing of contact lenses is not advisable. However, interactions with certain eye drops are possible, so you must ask your ophthalmologist what is recommended in your case (*Chapter 5* and *Chapter 6*).

⃝22 Can I take a plane or practice sports if I have glaucoma?

Yes. There is no danger in taking a plane or using any other form of transportation, and practicing sports is recommended as it causes intraocular pressure to drop. However, sports that require excessive exertion (such as weight lifting) or exercise that demands postures with the head down (yoga) are to be avoided, especially in advanced glaucoma, as they can cause intraocular pressure to rise. Vigorous physical activity is also not advisable in cases of pigmentary glaucoma (*Chapter 6*).

⃝23 Can stress, sexual relations or activities requiring intense use of the eyes aggravate glaucoma?

No. Stress, sexual relations and activities requiring intense use of the eyes are not risk factors in glaucoma and have no impact on the disease. People with glaucoma can, as a result, lead a completely normal life (*Chapter 3* and *Chapter 6*).

(24) Can glaucoma cause cataracts?

No. Glaucoma does not cause cataracts. However, it is not uncommon for someone with glaucoma to develop a cataract as well, as both diseases mainly affect people age 40 or older. Cataract surgery is usually not dangerous in people with glaucoma and may in fact lower intraocular pressure slightly (*Chapter 6*).

(25) Should I quit smoking if I have glaucoma?

Though it has not been established beyond any doubt that smoking is a risk factor in glaucoma, several recent studies have shown an association between glaucoma and smoking. It is thus best not to smoke (*Chapter 3*).

CHAPTER 1

UNDERSTANDING GLAUCOMA

Glaucoma affects one to three percent of the population of the Western world age 40 and over. The prevalence increases with age, reaching 10 percent among those over the age of 80. An estimated 400,000 Canadians have glaucoma. According to the World Health Organization, glaucoma is the second leading cause of blindness in the world, after cataracts. It is an extremely insidious disease that can destroy the functional capacity of the eye irreversibly and without warning. Though the incidence of glaucoma is high, the disease remains undetected in about half of those who have it, as it is painless (except in the rare cases of acute angle-closure glaucoma attack) and does not noticeably affect vision in the early stages. Screening is thus a major issue in the fight against glaucoma, especially as there are very effective treatments that can prevent or slow progression of the disease.

WHAT IS GLAUCOMA?

Glaucoma is a chronic eye disease that results in damage to the optic nerve. The damage is caused by several factors. Abnormally high pressure inside the eye is a key risk factor, but it is not the only one. Glaucoma is a disease that progresses slowly but gradually. As it damages the optic nerve, over time there is a loss of peripheral (side) vision and then, later, central vision as well. There are several types of glaucoma, with two main forms: open-angle glaucoma, the most frequent form of the disease; and angle-closure glaucoma (see *Chapter 2*). The "angle" is that formed by the iris and the cornea, also called the iridocorneal angle. This is the site of the drainage system, the trabecular meshwork, which controls pressure in the eye. Glaucoma can be treated by drops, laser therapy or surgery, depending on the type of glaucoma and its severity. Other forms of glaucoma include borderline glaucoma (glaucoma suspect) and pediatric or childhood glaucoma (see *Chapter 2*).

Glaucoma cannot be cured. However, like diabetes or high blood pressure, it can be controlled. Left untreated, glaucoma can eventually cause a narrowing of the visual field ("tunnel" vision) or partial or complete loss of sight. It is thus crucial that glaucoma be diagnosed early and its treatment started as soon as possible to slow or arrest its progression.

THE MECHANISM OF GLAUCOMATOUS DAMAGE

Glaucoma is characterized by damage to the optic nerve, called glaucomatous damage. The damage is often caused by increased pressure inside the eye (called intraocular pressure or IOP) (*Figure* ❶).

In the most common form of the disease, open-angle glaucoma, the rise in intraocular pressure is painless and is caused by poor drainage of the aqueous humour (a fluid that circulates in the front part of the eye) through the trabecular meshwork, which has become less permeable. As a result, the optic nerve is gradually destroyed and vision is lost.

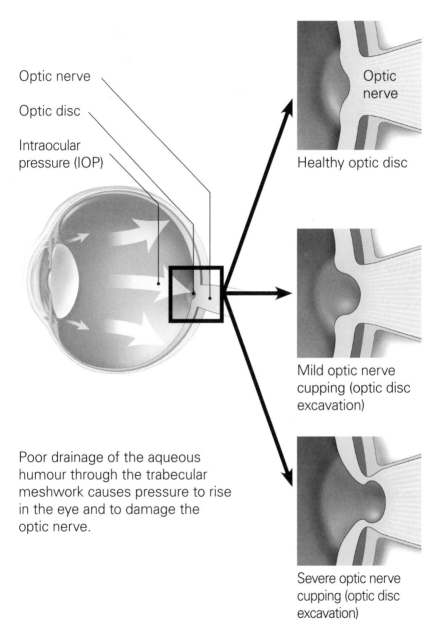

Optic nerve

Optic disc

Intraocular
pressure (IOP)

Optic
nerve

Healthy optic disc

Mild optic nerve
cupping (optic disc
excavation)

Poor drainage of the aqueous
humour through the trabecular
meshwork causes pressure to rise
in the eye and to damage the
optic nerve.

Severe optic nerve
cupping (optic disc
excavation)

❶ The mechanism of glaucomatous damage

In the much less common form of the disease, angle-closure glaucoma, intraocular pressure rises gradually with closure of the iridocorneal angle. When the trabecular meshwork is completely obstructed by the iris, intraocular pressure rises rapidly to very high levels. This is called an acute angle-closure glaucoma attack. Such attacks often cause violent eye pain and rapid vision loss. Emergency treatment is required.

These two main forms of glaucoma can be caused by a variety of medical disorders or by a predisposition to a particular type of glaucoma (see *Chapter 2*).

In most cases, people with glaucoma experience no symptoms that might lead them to suspect they have the disease.

HOW THE EYE WORKS

A brief explanation of how the eye works will help in understanding how glaucoma affects vision.

The eye is a spherical organ about 2.5 centimetres (1 inch) in diameter consisting of several covering layers plus internal structures (*Figure* ❷). Only part of the eye is visible; the rest is hidden inside the skull, in the eye socket. The eye is often said to work like a camera: to get a clear, crisp image, the diaphragm opens and closes to let in the right amount of light. The same principle applies to the eye. The image is focused by the cornea and the lens, and the iris serves as the diaphragm. The image thus formed is projected onto the retina, a thin membrane lining the back of the eye like film in a traditional roll-film camera.

The sclera and the conjunctiva

The sclera (the white of the eye) is the tough outer wall that surrounds and protects the eye. The optic nerve is attached to the sclera at the very back of the eye. The visible part of the sclera is covered by a thin, transparent membrane, the conjunctiva, which folds forward to become the lining of the inside of the eyelid.

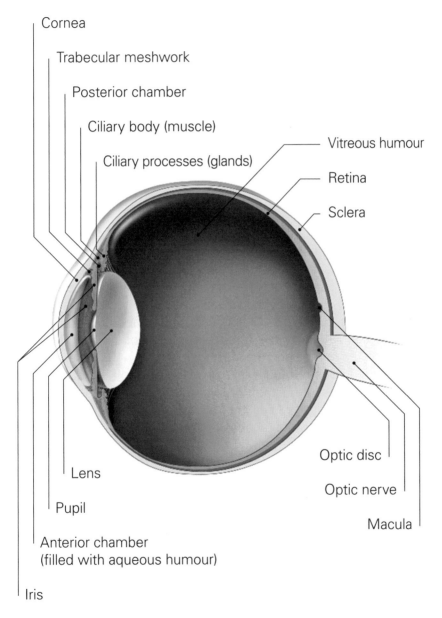

Cornea

Trabecular meshwork

Posterior chamber

Ciliary body (muscle)

Ciliary processes (glands)

Vitreous humour

Retina

Sclera

Lens

Optic disc

Optic nerve

Pupil

Macula

Anterior chamber
(filled with aqueous humour)

Iris

❷ Cross section of the eye

The cornea

The cornea is the transparent membrane at the front of the eye. It covers the eye like the glass that covers the face of a watch. About a half millimetre thick, the cornea forms a clear dome over the iris, from which it is separated by a fluid called the aqueous humour. The cornea controls the entry of light, protecting the inside of the eye by partially blocking ultraviolet rays. The thickness of the cornea is crucial information for interpreting intraocular pressure readings, as such readings may be higher than the actual pressure in people with thicker corneas. Conversely, those with thin corneas may show artificially low intraocular pressure readings.

Aqueous humour

The aqueous humour is a transparent fluid that flows between the iris and the lens, escaping through the pupil into the anterior chamber of the eye. It provides nutrition for the cornea, iris and lens. Composed essentially of water and nutrients, the aqueous humour is produced by the ciliary processes, glands located behind the iris. The aqueous humour is continuously filtered and drained into the venous circulation by the trabecular meshwork, a filter located between the cornea and the iris (*Figure* ❸).

The aqueous humour plays an important role in maintaining intraocular pressure. When it does not drain properly, generally because the drainage filter (the trabecular meshwork) is blocked, the accumulation of fluid causes intraocular pressure to rise and glaucoma to develop.

The trabecular meshwork and the uveoscleral pathway

The aqueous humour flows out of the eye along two pathways: the trabecular meshwork, the conventional outflow pathway; and the uveoscleral pathway, a secondary route through which 10 to 15 percent of the total flow drains.

The trabecular meshwork is a filter composed of fibres. It is located at the junction of the peripheral cornea and the iris (the iridocorneal angle). Its role is to filter aqueous humour outflow from

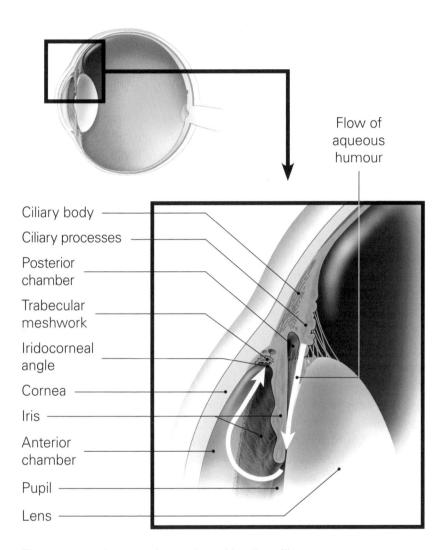

Flow of aqueous humour

Ciliary body

Ciliary processes

Posterior chamber

Trabecular meshwork

Iridocorneal angle

Cornea

Iris

Anterior chamber

Pupil

Lens

The aqueous humour is produced by the ciliary processes, located behind the iris. It flows from the posterior chamber through the pupil into the anterior chamber and then drains out of the eye through the trabecular meshwork, which lies in the iridocorneal angle.

❸ Flow of aqueous humour in the eye

the eye via the canal of Schlemm, a vein-like structure located behind the trabecular meshwork. In so doing, it controls pressure within the eye so that the globe of the eye retains its shape. Glaucoma develops when the trabecular meshwork malfunctions, causing pressure to build up in the eye.

A small but significant quantity of aqueous humour can exit the eye directly through the iris (anterior uvea), flowing to the choroid (a layer of the wall of the eye between the sclera and the retina) and the sclera. This is known as the uveoscleral outflow pathway. Unfortunately, this pathway cannot compensate for obstruction of the normal outflow pathway through the trabecular meshwork. The role of the uveoscleral pathway has not been clearly established, but scientists have discovered that it can account for more than 50 percent of total aqueous humour drainage in young monkeys (but only 10 percent in aging monkeys). This discovery has generated hope that one day it might be possible to modify this pathway in humans to increase aqueous humour through it and thus reduce intraocular pressure.

The iris and the pupil

The iris is the visible coloured part of the eye. At its centre is an opening, the pupil, which allows light to enter the eye and reach the retina. Like the aperture in a camera, the iris controls the amount of light entering the eye depending on the ambient lighting. The pupil contracts and dilates to regulate the amount of light that reaches the retina. In some cases, glaucoma develops because pupil dilation causes the iris to block the trabecular meshwork.

The lens

The lens is located behind the iris. The role of the lens is to focus images projected onto the back of the eye. To do this, the lens changes shape depending on the distance between the eye and the object viewed. The lens is held in place by ligaments (zonules of Zinn) that are connected to a muscle (the ciliary body).

With age, the lens grows larger, loses its flexibility and cannot change shape as easily. This results in presbyopia, a condition in which the eye loses its ability to focus on near objects. An enlarged lens can lead to angle-closure glaucoma in people predisposed to it, the enlarging lens pushing the iris forward and blocking the trabecular meshwork.

Vitreous humour

Between the lens and the retina, the eye is filled with a transparent gelatinous substance (like the white of an egg) called the vitreous humour, the vitreous body or the vitreous. The vitreous occupies about 80 percent of the volume of the eyeball. It is transparent, allowing light to travel to the retina, and it also transports nutrients important for the health of the eye.

The retina

The retina is a thin film of nerve tissue lining 75 percent of the inner surface of the eyeball. Here is where the photoreceptors are located, the cells that convert light to nerve impulses delivered to the brain by the nerve fibres of the optic nerve. A number of different retina examinations are used in people with glaucoma to assess nerve fibre loss.

The retina contains two types of photoreceptors (rods and cones), and each plays a different role in the perception of images.

There are approximately 120 million rods in each eye, and they are sensitive to dim light, allowing us to see at night. During the day, or in bright light, the rods stop responding. Rods cannot resolve fine detail or distinguish colours, but they are responsible for peripheral vision.

There are fewer cones (five million), but their capacity to distinguish detail is one hundred times greater than that of the rods. Very numerous in the macula, cones are responsible for colour vision and are used mainly in bright light (during the day or with artificial lighting). Cones are tuned to different portions of the colour spectrum: some perceive blue, others red and still others green. The cones are responsible for fine detail vision.

The macula

The macula is a very small area (about two millimetres in diameter) at the centre of the retina. The macula transmits 90 percent of the visual information processed by the brain. Composed of closely packed photoreceptor cells, the macula is responsible for fine detail vision (such as reading and recognizing faces) as well as colour detection. The retina as a whole allows us to see the book on the table, for example, but the macula makes it possible for us to read the words in the book. The macula is also called the "yellow spot" because of its yellow colour, due to a high concentration of lutein, an antioxidant of the carotenoid family. A number of different macula examinations are used in people with glaucoma to assess nerve fibre loss.

Retinal ganglion cells

Retinal ganglion cells form the innermost layer of the retina. These cells are nerve fibres that receive visual information from photoreceptors (cells sensitive to light) and transmit the information to the brain through the optic nerve. These ganglion cells die when glaucoma develops, and this is what causes the vision loss. The vision loss is permanent, as retinal ganglion cells do not regenerate. However, the loss of ganglion cells varies from one person to the next: some people do not experience a major loss despite elevated intraocular pressure, whereas others lose cells despite normal intraocular pressure.

The optic nerve

There are two optic nerves, one at the back of each eye. These nerves transmit visual information to the brain. At birth, each optic nerve is composed of roughly one million nerve fibres that stretch from the ganglion cells of the retina out the eyeball through the lamina cribrosa into the brain. The number of nerve fibres in each optic nerve decreases with age, as there is an average loss of five thousand fibres per year. In glaucoma, the pace of this gradual loss of fibres of the optic nerve accelerates.

Optic nerve head

The optic nerve head, or optic disc, is the visible part of the optic nerve. It is about 1.5 mm in diameter and is located on the retina where the optic fibres of the retinal ganglion cells meet. Glaucoma severity is evaluated from the extent of the damage to the optic nerve head—which is determined by measuring optic nerve cupping (or optic disc excavation), that is, the size of the empty space created by loss of optic nerve fibre. To assess the extent of the nerve damage, doctors measure the diameter of the empty space, or excavation, and compare it to the diameter of the nerve head.

Lamina cribrosa

The lamina cribrosa is the part of the sclera where optic nerve fibres carrying visual information from the retina to the brain exit the eye. The lamina cribrosa plays a key role in glaucoma. Studies of the morphology of the lamina cribrosa demonstrate that if it is not rigid enough it will bulge too much in response to changes in intraocular pressure, causing damage to optic nerve fibres. This explains why some people get glaucoma even though their intraocular pressure remains low.

HOW WE SEE

Light passes first through the cornea, the aqueous humour, the lens and the vitreous humour before falling on the retina. It is there, not in the brain, that processing of the image by the nervous system begins. In fact, many anatomists consider the retina an extension of the brain. As thin as a sheet of paper, the retina is nonetheless more complex and more sensitive than photographic film. It has ten distinct layers, each with a specific function. Light must cross several of these layers to reach the 125 million photoreceptors (light-sensitive cells) that absorb the light and convert it to nerve impulses, which are relayed to the brain via the optic nerve.

CHAPTER 2
FORMS AND
SYMPTOMS

Excluding borderline glaucoma (glaucoma suspect) and childhood glaucoma (see below in this chapter), there are two main forms of glaucoma: open-angle glaucoma and angle-closure glaucoma. The "angle" referred to is the iridocorneal angle, formed by the junction of the iris and the cornea.

Many factors can lead to obstruction or closure of the iridocorneal angle, everything from an anatomical condition to disease, accident or genetic predisposition. These factors define the different types of glaucoma in each of its main forms. Factors can coexist, however, and it is sometimes difficult to decide which type of glaucoma a patient has. In fact, some people have several types of glaucoma at once. Also, the type of glaucoma a patient has may change over time.

A WORD ABOUT SYMPTOMS

Both main forms of glaucoma generally affect both eyes at once, though not always to the same extent. Certain types of glaucoma can, however, affect only one eye, particularly angle-closure glaucoma, exfoliative glaucoma and post-traumatic glaucoma. In both open-angle glaucoma and angle-closure glaucoma, there is damage to the optic nerve (and, as a result, loss of visual field), which can lead to blindness. In both open-angle and angle-closure glaucoma, the gradual destruction of optic nerve fibre is painless. The eye appears normal and there is no vision loss in the early stages, unless intraocular pressure increases rapidly and dramatically, as in the case of an acute angle-closure glaucoma attack (see *Primary angle-closure glaucoma* below in this chapter), but in the end, vision is affected. The optic nerve fibres are like telephone lines that connect different parts of the eye to the brain. The death of these fibres leads to a progressive loss of visual field, starting with peripheral (side) vision and gradually affecting central vision as well. In very advanced glaucoma, the patient has the impression that he or she is looking through a tunnel and that the tunnel is gradually getting narrower and narrower. The problem is that there can be substantial optic nerve fibre loss before any symptoms appear. According to one study, up to 40 percent of the nerve fibres of the optic nerve can be destroyed without any loss of visual field. In addition, the vision loss is hard for the patient to detect, as it is very gradual. Only one eye may be affected and the other may compensate, and central vision (what we use the most) is not affected right away. This is why so many people do not notice the visual field loss until 70 to 80 percent of their optic nerve fibres are destroyed.

The only hope, then, of early detection of glaucoma is regular eye examinations. The Canadian Ophthalmological Society recommends that people at risk for glaucoma or with a family history of glaucoma have complete eye examinations at least every three years if they are over age 40 and at least once a year if they are over age 65.

GLAUCOMA SUSPECT

As the name suggests, a glaucoma suspect is a patient suspected of having open-angle or angle-closure glaucoma because he or she shows signs of glaucoma or has one or more glaucoma risk factors yet there is no optic nerve damage or vision loss.

Signs observed in open-angle glaucoma suspects include elevated intraocular pressure without optic nerve damage or visual field defect and suspicious cupping of the optic disc (head of the optic nerve) without elevated intraocular pressure.

Risk factors that could lead to classification as a glaucoma suspect include family history of glaucoma, elevated intraocular pressure (ocular hypertension), pseudoexfoliative syndrome, pigment dispersion syndrome, uveitis, a suspicious optic disc and/or visual field and eye trauma (see below in this chapter and *Chapter 3*).

Glaucoma suspects also include people with a narrow iridocorneal angle. Because of the anatomy of the eye in such people, there is risk that the iridocorneal angle will close. People who are hyperopic (farsighted) in particular are likely to have shallow anterior chambers (between the iris and the cornea), as are people whose lenses have grown with age or due to a cataract. Such people are angle-closure glaucoma suspects.

Long-term monitoring of glaucoma suspects is the only way to know for sure if glaucoma is present. To check if the optic nerve is damaged and to assess the extent of the damage, the doctor measures the diameter of the empty space created by optic nerve fibre loss, what is known as optic disc cupping or optic nerve cupping. If the size of the "cup" grows from one visit to the next, then a diagnosis of glaucoma may be made. However, some people are born with larger than average cups, in which case the optic nerve looks glaucomatous. As long as there is no progression in the size of the cup in a patient without other symptoms (such as a visual field deficit), the patient will continue to be considered a glaucoma suspect.

The ophthalmologist may nonetheless decide to initiate treatment in case of one or more risk factors, such as very elevated intraocular pressure, very pronounced optic nerve cupping and a family history of glaucoma.

PRIMARY OPEN-ANGLE GLAUCOMA

Glaucoma is said to be primary when it is not due to another eye disease. Open-angle means that the opening of the iridocorneal angle is normal, which is not the case with angle-closure glaucoma (*Figure* ❶).

Primary open-angle glaucoma is asymptomatic in the early stages, that is, neither the person who has the disease nor his or her friends and family will notice any signs or symptoms.

The goal of treatment (drug therapy, laser procedure or surgery) is to lower and stabilize intraocular pressure.

There are two types of primary open-angle glaucoma: high-tension primary open-angle glaucoma and normal-tension glaucoma.

High-tension primary open-angle glaucoma

This type of glaucoma, also called chronic open-angle glaucoma, affects people with elevated intraocular pressure (more than 21 millimeters of mercury or mm Hg). High-tension primary open-angle glaucoma accounts for 60 to 70 percent of all cases of glaucoma diagnosed in Europe and North America (it is less common in Asia). This type of glaucoma generally develops in people over age 50, and its frequency has a strong tendency to increase with age.

Often intraocular pressure is only slightly elevated in high-tension primary open-angle glaucoma (between 21 and 30 mm Hg), but it can run as high as 30 to 50 mm in some cases. When making the diagnosis, the ophthalmologist must ensure there are no other risk factors (pigment dispersion syndrome, pseudoexfoliation syndrome, etc.) that would suggest a diagnosis of secondary open-angle glaucoma.

In addition to elevated intraocular pressure, patients with high tension primary open-angle glaucoma often present fluctuations in intraocular pressure. When the fluctuations are substantial, damage to the optic nerve may result.

In patients with high-tension primary open-angle glaucoma, the elevated intraocular pressure stems from poor aqueous humour

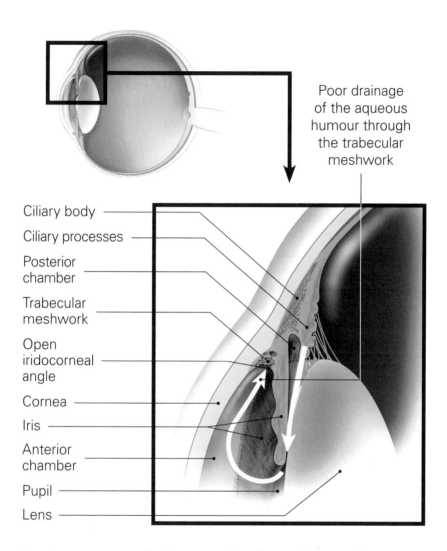

Poor drainage of the aqueous humour through the trabecular meshwork

Ciliary body

Ciliary processes

Posterior chamber

Trabecular meshwork

Open iridocorneal angle

Cornea

Iris

Anterior chamber

Pupil

Lens

In primary open-angle glaucoma, the elevated intraocular pressure stems from poor drainage of the aqueous humour from the eye, even if examination of the trabecular meshwork shows no obstacles to evacuation.

❶ Primary open-angle glaucoma

drainage, even if examination of the trabecular meshwork shows no obstacles to evacuation through this pathway. This dysfunction is age-related, as the trabecular meshwork becomes less permeable with age. However, specialists believe there are other reasons for poor aqueous humour drainage that are still not well understood.

Normal-tension glaucoma

About 30 percent of patients with primary open-angle glaucoma do not have elevated intraocular pressure. This is called normal-tension glaucoma. In normal-tension glaucoma, there is glaucomatous damage but intraocular pressure is normal in repeated pressure measurements and the iridocorneal angle is open. Intraocular pressure measurements can, however, be affected by a thick cornea, severe astigmatism (vision impairment due to a defect in the curvature of the cornea) or an irregular corneal surface. This means that real intraocular pressure can sometimes be underestimated or overestimated.

In addition, intraocular pressure may be normal at the time of the visit to the ophthalmologist but elevated at other times of the day. In fact, major fluctuations in intraocular pressure are characteristic of people with glaucoma, with fluctuations of 12 mm or more over the course of a day in people with untreated glaucoma compared to 5 mm in those without the disease. This means that what may look like normal-tension glaucoma at the time of a visit to the ophthalmologist could turn out to be another form of glaucoma. The ophthalmologist may ask the patient to measure his or her pressure throughout the day to check whether it is higher at certain times of the day.

As it is hard to differentiate between normal-tension and high-tension primary open-angle glaucoma on the basis of intraocular pressure measurements, other risk factors must be identified. In some cases, the patient has a history of elevated intraocular pressure that damaged the optic nerve but later returned to normal. This is seen in particular in people who have experienced an eye trauma, pigment dispersion or eye inflammation, or have used cortisone and then discontinued it. In such cases, the normal-tension glaucoma is not considered a chronic disease but rather the result of an event. The patient is then followed for some time until the ophthalmologist is sure the damage is not progressing. The glaucomatous damage remains irreversible, but the patient no longer needs monitoring or treatment.

In other cases, the optic nerve and the ganglion cells are more sensitive to normal intraocular pressures for genetic reasons. The ophthalmologist also looks for factors that could damage the blood vessels of the retina, leading to poor oxygenation of the optic nerve (diabetes, for example, or certain medications), or for vascular factors, such as atherosclerosis (a disorder that leads to clogging of the arteries and disruption of blood flow), ocular perfusion pressure (difference between systemic blood pressure and intraocular pressure), a thin cornea or vasospasms (sudden, transient constriction of a blood vessel).

A scientific study has shown that when intraocular pressure is reduced by at least 30 percent in patients presenting normal-tension glaucoma, disease progression can be controlled.

SECONDARY OPEN-ANGLE GLAUCOMA

Glaucoma is considered secondary when it results from another eye disease, an injury, eye surgery or even certain medical treatments.

As in primary open-angle glaucoma, the goal of treatment (drug therapy, laser procedure or surgery) is to lower and stabilize intraocular pressure.

Of the numerous types of secondary open-angle glaucomas, the main ones are described below.

Steroid-induced glaucoma

This type of glaucoma is caused by prolonged use of local or systemic corticosteroids to treat chronic, most often inflammatory, disorders. Local therapies (corticosteroid eye drops and intravitreal injections) cause the most rapid and the most dramatic increases in intraocular pressure. In some patients, this occurs because corticosteroids reduce the permeability of the trabecular meshwork.

Pigmentary glaucoma

Pigmentary glaucoma is caused by pigment dispersion syndrome. Not everyone with pigment dispersion syndrome develops glaucoma, but the probability is significantly greater.

In pigment dispersion syndrome, melanin particles accumulate in all parts of the eye where the aqueous humour circulates. Melanin is a pigment found in the iris and in the back of the eye, between the retina and the choroid. Pigment dispersion syndrome develops in people with a particular type of structure of the anterior chamber of the eye. Some people who are myopic, for example, have a concave iris that bulges backward, causing the back part of the iris to rub against the fibres that hold the lens in place (the zonules). This causes dispersion of pigment, which obstructs the trabecular meshwork and results in elevated intraocular pressure.

Pigment dispersion syndrome is more frequent in men than in women and occurs mainly between ages 20 and 50. With age, the iris loses its concavity, the rubbing diminishes and the pigment dispersion ceases. However, if the trabecular meshwork has suffered too much damage by this time, the elevated intraocular pressure may persist. In other cases, the glaucoma disappears.

The treatment for pigmentary glaucoma is similar to that used for primary open-angle glaucoma, but sometimes an iridotomy is performed in the early stages of the disease to try to reduce rubbing of the iris (see *Chapter 5*).

Exfoliative glaucoma

Exfoliative glaucoma is caused by pseudoexfoliation syndrome (PEX), which is often accompanied by pigment dispersion. PEX is characterized by deposits of whitish-grey protein and pigment on the anterior lens surface. Such deposits are also present in all parts of the eye irrigated by the aqueous humour and can accumulate in the trabecular meshwork, blocking drainage of the aqueous humour and provoking elevated intraocular pressure.

In addition, pseudoexfoliation weakens the lens zonules, the suspensory ligaments that hold the lens in place. The lens changes shape as a result. It becomes rounder and takes up more place in the eye, pushing the iris to the front of the eye, blocking the trabecular meshwork and provoking secondary angle-closure glaucoma. It is thus not exceptional for exfoliation syndrome and angle-closure glaucoma to occur together.

Not everyone with PEX develops glaucoma, but the risk is greater. In addition, people with PEX tend to experience major fluctuations in intraocular pressure, which means closer ophthalmological monitoring is often required.

Post-traumatic glaucoma

This form of glaucoma sometimes develops many years after an eye injury. It stems from sequelae of damage to the iridocorneal angle tissue and the aqueous humour drainage system. Anyone who has had an eye injury should be followed regularly in ophthalmology or optometry for the rest of his or her life to watch for development of glaucoma.

Uveitic glaucoma

Secondary glaucoma can sometimes accompany or follow uveitis (inflammation of the interior of the eye). Uveitis generally causes intraocular pressure to drop, but some types of uveitis cause it to rise. In addition, cortisone is sometimes used to treat the inflammation, and cortisone is known to cause intraocular pressure to rise.

Uveitic glaucoma can take the form of open-angle glaucoma, with a risk of eventually turning into angle-closure glaucoma as the inflammatory cells multiply around the iridocorneal angle and cause the iris to fuse to the trabecular meshwork.

Neovascular glaucoma

Neovascular glaucoma can develop in response to severe, chronic ischemia (insufficient blood supply) in the retina (retinal ischemia). Retinal ischemia can be triggered by diseases such as diabetic retinopathy, which affects people with diabetes, or it may be associated with retinal vein occlusion (see *Chapter 3*). Neovessels (new abnormal blood vessels) and fibrous tissue invade the iridocorneal angle, preventing drainage of the aqueous humour and causing intraocular pressure to rise.

People with open-angle glaucoma are unusually susceptible to retinal vein occlusion, which can be accompanied by ischemia. In this case, the open-angle glaucoma turns into neovascular glaucoma.

With time, the neovessels in the iridocorneal angle may contract and close the angle, causing secondary angle-closure glaucoma.

Neovascular glaucoma is treated by treating the underlying disease. Retinal ischemia is often treated by injections of antiangiogenics (anti-VEGFs) or laser therapy (see *Chapter 5*). Laser therapy can be more difficult, however, when the neovascular growth in the iridocorneal angle is of long date and the angle is closed and scarred.

PRIMARY ANGLE-CLOSURE GLAUCOMA

This form of glaucoma is not as common (10 to 20 percent of all cases of glaucoma), except among Asians and Inuit. It is also more serious, as an acute angle-closure glaucoma attack can very quickly lead to blindness. This type of glaucoma is characterized by a narrower than normal iridocorneal angle. With time, this angle may become even narrower and may close, completely or partially obstructing the trabecular meshwork (*Figure* ❷). Complete obstruction of the meshwork can trigger an acute angle-closure glaucoma attack, with a very dramatic and extremely painful increase in intraocular pressure. In addition to sudden pain in the eyes, such an attack can cause nausea and rapid deterioration of vision. This is a medical emergency. Without rapid treatment, blindness will occur quickly.

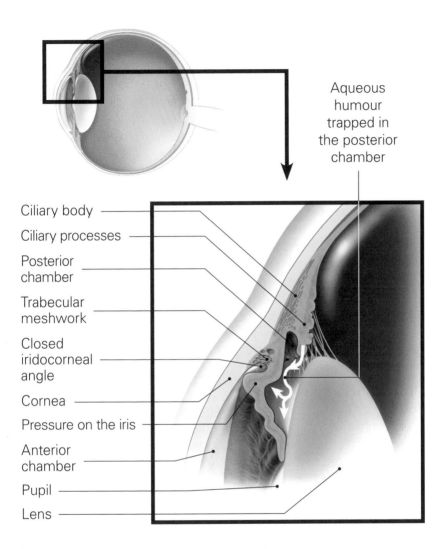

Aqueous humour trapped in the posterior chamber

Ciliary body

Ciliary processes

Posterior chamber

Trabecular meshwork

Closed iridocorneal angle

Cornea

Pressure on the iris

Anterior chamber

Pupil

Lens

In angle-closure glaucoma with pupillary block, the aqueous humour can no longer flow through the pupil from the posterior to the anterior chamber. As a result, the iris is forced into the trabecular meshwork (the eye's drain) and obstructs it.

❷ Primary angle-closure glaucoma with pupillary block

It is, accordingly, best to prevent such attacks by screening during comprehensive eye health examinations, by regular monitoring, by avoiding certain drugs and possibly by preventive iridotomy (see *Chapter 5*). However, 50 to 60 percent of people with primary angle-closure glaucoma never have an acute angle-closure glaucoma attack or even present any symptoms.

Angle closure can be caused by a pupillary block, iris plateau syndrome or a ciliary block.

Pupillary block

Angle closure most often results from a pupillary block, that is, the anterior surface of the lens seals against the pupil and blocks the flow of aqueous humour to the anterior chamber of the eye. The result is pressure on the iris, forcing it toward the cornea and closing the iridocorneal angle (*Figure* ❷ above in this chapter).

People with hypermetropia are particularly predisposed to pupillary blockage because their eyes are small, and the structures of their eyes are thus very close together. Pupillary block is often genetic and is common among Asians and Inuit.

Plateau iris syndrome

The key characteristic of eyes with plateau iris syndrome is the prominent ciliary processes (glands that produce the aqueous humour), which are anteriorly positioned (rotated forward) instead of being directed to the inside of the eye. This anatomical anomaly puts pressure on the iris, crowding it against the cornea and causing partial or total closure of the iridocorneal angle over time. Fortunately, angle closure does not develop in everyone with plateau iris syndrome, but such patients must be monitored.

Ciliary block

This very rare form of glaucoma can be caused by an anatomical predisposition but is mainly due to intraocular surgery. In this form of glaucoma, the iris is pushed against the lens due to an anterior rotation of the ciliary body (part of the eye composed of the ciliary processes arranged in a circle forming a frill where the choroid meets the iris). As a result, the aqueous humour flows from the posterior chamber to the vitreous cavity instead of to the anterior chamber. The iris and the lens are thus pushed forward, blocking the iridocorneal angle. The recommended treatment is pupil dilation. Laser or surgical therapy may also be required.

SECONDARY ANGLE-CLOSURE GLAUCOMA

Various eye diseases can cause angle closure by pulling or pushing the iris forward, leading to secondary angle-closure glaucoma. This can happen in particular when the lens becomes swollen or displaced as a result of any number of disorders. The lens then exerts pressure on the iris, which in turn obstructs the trabecular meshwork. Other causes include eye trauma or eye surgery. Tumours in the back of the eye can also cause angle closure, as can cysts in the iris or the ciliary body. These disorders put pressure on the iris, which then obstructs the trabecular meshwork.

No matter what the cause of secondary angle-closure glaucoma, the goal of treatment is to prevent complete angle closure, generally by suppressing whatever is contributing to the closure. A laser procedure (iridotomy) is often required. In some cases, cataract surgery or vitrectomy (surgical removal of the vitreous body) will be suggested to the patient. It is very common for secondary angle-closure glaucoma to turn into primary open-angle glaucoma after surgery if the iris has seriously damaged the trabecular meshwork.

GLAUCOMA IN CHILDREN

Glaucoma is much less common among children than among adults. It can, however, appear in the very first days of life or later. Childhood glaucoma can occur without any known cause, or it may be caused by a congenital malformation or a syndrome. When the glaucoma is not associated with a malformation or syndrome, it is called congenital or juvenile glaucoma. Not all the genes involved in these forms of glaucoma have yet been identified. Glaucoma in children is considered secondary when it arises as a result of certain events, such as an eye trauma, an inflammation or a tumour. All forms of childhood glaucoma present the same signs and symptoms as adult glaucoma, with the addition of other symptoms in the case of congenital glaucoma. As in adults, the elevation of intraocular pressure can damage the optic nerve, leading to vision disorders or even loss of sight if left untreated.

Drug treatments are used mainly to complement surgery. In fact, surgery is less risky in children than in adults, and side effects from eye drops are more frequent among children. There are actually eye drops used only in children. As for surgery, some procedures are specific to children (trabeculotomy, for example, which involves creating an opening in the trabecular meshwork so the aqueous humour can flow normally), while others are similar to those recommended in adults. Laser treatments used in adults, however, are rarely used with children.

Glaucoma related to a malformation or a syndrome

This type of glaucoma can develop at any age, even in adults. These eye malformations and syndromes, hereditary or not, obstruct aqueous humour outflow. They include aniridia, Lowe syndrome, Sturge-Weber syndrome, autosomal dominant iris hypoplasia, iridogoniodysgenesis and Peters anomaly. The glaucoma that results from these malformations or syndromes can be open-angle or angle-closure glaucoma.

Congenital glaucoma

Though congenital glaucoma is the most common type of glaucoma in children, it is still rare (one in 10,000 births). Onset is generally between birth and three years of age. In addition to the usual symptoms seen in adults, there are other noticeable symptoms, such as excessive tearing, light sensitivity (photophobia) and eyelid closure on exposure to light (blepharospasm).

Juvenile glaucoma

Juvenile glaucoma occurs in older children and adolescents, generally in families with a history of similar glaucoma. Systematic screening for the disease is thus justified in these "at risk" families. However, we do not yet know all the genetic mutations at the origin of this form of glaucoma.

Secondary glaucoma in children

Secondary glaucoma can develop following eye inflammation, trauma, tumour or surgery for a congenital cataract. Uveitis (intraocular inflammation of the uvea, the part of the eye that includes the iris, the ciliary body and the choroid) is also a major cause of secondary glaucoma.

WHAT YOU NEED TO KNOW

- Glaucoma is associated with eye pressure that is too high for your eye.
- There are two main forms of glaucoma: open-angle glaucoma and angle-closure glaucoma.
- Open-angle glaucoma and angle-closure glaucoma share certain features:
    - Optic nerve fibres are destroyed.
    - There are few symptoms in the early stages.
    - There is a gradual loss of vision (beginning with peripheral vision) that is hard to detect.
    - Vision loss cannot be recovered.
    - The only way to prevent serious vision loss is early detection.
- There is also an acute form of angle-closure glaucoma, characterized by a rapid and very dramatic increase in intraocular pressure. Such angle-closure glaucoma attacks cause sudden, severe pain in the eyes, nausea and rapid vision deterioration.

ONE PERSON'S STORY

Name: John	**Age:** 69 years old

Occupation: Retired

John has been enjoying cultural outings since his retirement. It was during one such outing, while watching a film, that he felt a sudden pain in his eyes and his vision went blurry. The symptoms quickly got worse, so much so that he had to leave the movie theatre. His wife, who was with him, drove him immediately to the emergency room at the nearest hospital. On the way to the hospital, the pain in John's eyes was excruciating, and he was seeing coloured halos around the lights along the highway. The emergency-room doctor who examined him immediately diagnosed an acute angle-closure glaucoma attack and rapidly called in an ophthalmologist. The ophthalmologist placed drops in John's eyes to lower his intra-ocular pressure (IOP), which was very elevated (62 mm Hg). In fact, there was a risk of major damage to the optic nerve and an irreversible loss of sight. The ophthalmologist performed a laser procedure in both eyes to allow the aqueous humour to circulate freely once again and thus lower the intra-ocular pressure. John was able to leave the hospital that same day. His vision gradually improved in the days following his visit to the hospital and not long after was completely restored in both eyes.

John feels lucky. He knows that if the attack had not been treated quickly, he could have gone blind in both eyes. He now has to see an ophthalmologist once a year to make sure his intraocular pressure is not increasing again.

CHAPTER 3
RISK FACTORS

The genes and mechanisms responsible for glaucoma have not all been identified. As a result, we do not yet know the exact causes of glaucoma. However, we do know that the development of glaucoma is promoted by the presence of a number of risk factors (elevated eye pressure being the most common) and their effects tend to be cumulative. Of the other risk factors, some are recognized but others are more controversial, as study results are sometimes contradictory. At any rate, a number of known risk factors can be modified by treatment or changes in lifestyle to preserve the sight of people with glaucoma or those at high risk of developing it.

KNOWN RISK FACTORS

Intraocular pressure (IOP)

Intraocular pressure (IOP) is recognized as one of the main risk factors in primary open-angle glaucoma.

However, elevated intraocular pressure is not the only glaucoma risk factor. In fact, 30 percent of people with glaucoma have normal or low intraocular pressure (see *Normal-tension glaucoma* in *Chapter 2*), a clear indication of other problems. In addition, some people have elevated intraocular pressure but do not have glaucoma (see *Glaucoma suspect* in *Chapter 2*). One reason for this is that intraocular pressure can fluctuate substantially over the course of a day, which means measurements obtained may depend on the time of day they are taken. Intraocular pressure can rise even when lying down. It can also rise gradually with age. The rigidity of the cornea, which depends mainly on its thickness, must also be considered (see *Measuring intraocular pressure [IOP]* and *Measuring the thickness of the cornea* in *Chapter 4*).

Intraocular pressure alone, without consideration of these other variables, is not enough for a diagnosis of glaucoma.

WHAT IS NORMAL INTRAOCULAR PRESSURE?

In adults, intraocular pressure is generally between 8 and 21 mm Hg (millimetres of mercury), with an average of 15.5 mm Hg and pressure about the same in both eyes. Intraocular pressure above 21 mm Hg is considered elevated.

Intraocular pressure is measured with a number of devices, the main one being the Goldmann tonometer. Other devices include the Tono-Pen, the Icare, Pascal and Perkins tonometers, the pneumotonometer, the air-pulse tonometer and the Ocular Response Analyser (ORA) (see *Measuring intraocular pressure [IOP]* in *Chapter 4*).

Age

Intraocular pressure can increase with age. Age is therefore an important risk factor, particularly in primary open-angle glaucoma (POAG). Most people with elevated intraocular pressure are over age 40, mainly because the trabecular meshwork becomes less permeable with age. The frequency of glaucoma increases with age, rising from two percent over age 40 to five percent over age 65 and 10 percent over age 80.

However, even children can get glaucoma (see *Chapter 2*).

Family history

Others with the disease are often found in the families of people with glaucoma—a father, mother, sister, brother, grandparent, uncle or aunt. Family history is a long-recognized risk factor in the open-angle as well as the angle-closure forms of glaucoma, but glaucoma can nonetheless occur spontaneously in people with no family history of the disease. A number of genes involved in glaucoma have been identified in the last decade, and studies show that when a member of the immediate family has glaucoma (father, mother, brother or sister), the risk of developing the disease is 20 percent. Regular consultation of an optometrist or an ophthalmologist is thus recommended when there is a family history of glaucoma, especially after age 40.

Prolonged use of corticosteroids

Prolonged use of corticosteroids, administered directly to the eyes or taken by mouth, can cause intraocular pressure to rise and trigger secondary open-angle glaucoma. Corticosteroid use can also lead to normal-tension glaucoma (see *Chapter 2*) if it causes damage to the optic nerve that is only discovered years later, when the patient is no longer using corticosteroids and intraocular pressure has returned to normal. The normal-tension glaucoma is then non-progressive.

Corticosteroids, sometimes called steroids, are medicines that mimic cortisone, a hormone that is present in the body but in much smaller quantities. Corticosteroids are used to treat rheumatoid arthritis, among other things, as well as certain eye inflammations. They are also used to help tolerate contact lenses.

It is recommended that people who use corticosteroids consult an optometrist or an ophthalmologist regularly to ensure that their intraocular pressure remains normal.

Note that inhaled corticosteroids taken for asthma, intranasal corticosteroids for allergic rhinitis and creams or ointments for eczema have little impact on glaucoma.

Pseudoexfoliative syndrome

Pseudoexfoliative syndrome (PEX) is a common factor in secondary open-angle or angle-closure glaucoma. It is characterized by whitish or grey deposits on the lens. This material, as well as pigment, is deposited on the trabecular meshwork, interfering with drainage of the aqueous humour. Glaucoma results in 15 percent of cases over five years.

Pigment dispersion syndrome

In pigment dispersion syndrome, the iris rubs against the lens and the zonules, causing loss of pigment from the back of the iris. This pigment is released into the anterior chamber of the eye and is deposited on the cornea, iris, lens and trabecular meshwork. The deposits on the trabecular meshwork provoke an increase in intraocular pressure. People with this syndrome have a 15 percent risk of developing secondary open-angle glaucoma over five years.

Eye injury

Glaucoma can develop following an injury or accident to the eye—getting hit in the eye by a hockey stick, for example. When the trabecular meshwork is damaged as a result of an eye injury, intraocular pressure rises, causing secondary open-angle glaucoma. The risk of developing elevated intraocular pressure is seven to eight percent in anyone with a major eye injury, even if intraocular pressure does not rise immediately after the accident. When eye injury causes swelling or displacement of the lens, it can trigger secondary angle-closure glaucoma.

Ethnicity

Primary open-angle glaucoma is the most common glaucoma in the West and in Africa. It accounts for 90 percent of all cases of glaucoma in Canada. Blacks, however, tend to develop more serious cases of primary open-angle glaucoma than Whites, and to develop it at an earlier age. Among Asians and Inuit, primary angle-closure glaucoma is decidedly more common than among Whites. Normal-tension glaucoma is also more frequent among Asians. We do not yet understand why ethnicity is a risk factor in glaucoma.

Myopia

Primary open-angle glaucoma is slightly more common among people with myopia than in the rest of the population, especially in high or severe myopia (8.00 diopters or more). The configuration of the optic nerve in people with high myopia makes them more vulnerable to fluctuations in intraocular pressure.

Pigmentary glaucoma (see *Chapter 2*) is also seen mainly in people with myopia. The iris, which is concave in myopia, rubs against the lens and the zonules (fibrous strands connecting the lens to the ciliary body). This rubbing action causes pigment to shed from the back of the iris, clogging the trabecular meshwork and causing intraocular pressure to rise.

WHAT IS A RISK FACTOR

A risk factor does not, in and of itself, cause a disease. Its presence increases the probability that the disease will develop, especially when other risk factors are present as well. However, the presence of risk factors is no guarantee that the disease will actually develop. In other words, several risk factors may be present, yet the disease may never develop. On the other hand, the disease may develop even when no risk factors are present.

Hyperopia (farsightedness)

Hyperopia (also called hypermetropia or farsightedness) is a risk factor in primary angle-closure glaucoma. This is because the eyes are smaller and more compact in people with hyperopia. With time, the lens grows and takes up more and more space in the anterior part of the eye, putting pressure on the iris, which eventually obstructs the trabecular meshwork.

Certain medications

Some medications can cause intraocular pressure to rise in certain people, leading to primary angle-closure glaucoma. Medications that can do this include anticholinergic drops (atropine, homatropine, cyclopentolate, tropicamide and scopolamine), drugs with anticholinergic properties (systemic atropine, antihistamines, antiparkinsonians, phenothiazine antipsychotics, intestinal antispasmodics, botulinum toxins such as Botox or topiramate and adrenergic drops such as those with phenylephrine, hydroxyamphetamine, epinephrine, dipivefrin, apraclonidine or cocaine) and drugs with adrenergic properties (vasoconstrictors, decongestants, CSN stimulants, bronchodilators and appetite depressants). Most of these drugs dilate the pupil, which causes obstruction of the trabecular meshwork by the iris in predisposed patients. Others cause edema (swelling) of the choroid, which pushes the lens and the iris onto the trabecular meshwork in some people with small eyes.

Injection of air or sulphur hexafluoride (SF_6) into the eyes after surgery or in case of surgical complication can also provoke secondary angle-closure glaucoma.

Retinal vein occlusion

Retinal vein occlusion is a disorder that mainly effects people with high blood pressure and atherosclerosis. It is caused by a sudden obstruction of venous circulation in the optic nerve and it can trigger open-angle glaucoma. In some cases where retinal vein occlusion is accompanied by ischemia (insufficient blood flow), new abnormal blood vessels (neovessels) and fibrovascular tissue will proliferate in the iris and in the iridocorneal angle, evenutally plugging the trabecular meshwork and causing neovascular glaucoma (see *Chapter 2*). Patients with open-angle glaucoma are also susceptible to retinal vein occlusion.

Eye anatomy

The anatomy of the eye is a risk factor in open-angle as well as angle-closure glaucoma. The closer together the structures of the eye, as in people with hyperopia (see *Hyperopia [farsightedness]* above in this chapter), the greater the risk of angle-closure glaucoma.

The structure of the optic nerve and the arrangement of its blood vessels probably play a role in the onset of primary open-angle glaucoma as well. In addition, the lamina cribrosa, through which the optic nerve passes on its way from the retina to the brain, is weaker in some people. Studies have shown that when the lamina cribrosa is not rigid enough it tends to move, damaging the fibres of the optic nerve. These two factors may explain why some people with low intraocular pressure nonetheless develop glaucoma.

Eye surgery

Any eye surgery can cause intraocular pressure to rise because of inflammation, anterior synechiae (adhesion of iris and corneal tissue), use of steroids or injury to the iridocorneal angle, and this can lead to secondary open-angle or closed glaucoma.

Sickle-cell anemia

In people with sickle-cell anemia (a common hereditary blood disorder), the red blood cells become rigid and assume a sickle shape. Should someone with sickle-cell anemia develop hyphema (blood in the anterior chamber of the eye, often caused by eye injury), the deformed red blood cells will have difficulty passing through the channels that drain the eye, which can cause intraocular pressure to rise and possibly secondary open-angle glaucoma—or even neovascular glaucoma in extreme cases (see *Chapter 2*).

Iridocorneal endothelial syndrome (ICE)

Iridocorneal endothelial syndrome (ICE) is a disorder of the cornea, in which a membrane forms behind the cornea. This membrane sometimes migrates to the trabecular meshwork and obstructs it, causing intraocular pressure to rise, which in turn may provoke secondary open-angle glaucoma (or secondary angle-closure glaucoma if the membrane contracts and pulls the iris into contact with the trabecular meshwork).

Intraocular tumours

Though fortunately relatively rare, intraocular tumours (such as choroidal melanoma or retinoblastoma) can cause glaucoma. Located under or in the retina, these tumours can cause secondary angle-closure glaucoma by pushing the iris and the lens towards the front of the eye. They can also cause neovascular glaucoma (see *Chapter 2*) by stimulating growth of abnormal blood vessels in the iridocorneal angle. In some cases, cancer cells migrate and clog the trabecular meshwork.

Inflammatory reactions

Iritis (inflammation of the iris), certain forms of arthritis and uveitis (inflammation of the uvea) can cause obstruction of the trabecular meshwork and trigger secondary open-angle or angle-closure glaucoma, or, in rare cases, neovascular glaucoma. In addition, people with arthritis sometimes take corticosteroids, which can further increase the risk.

Developmental anomalies

With certain rare congenital abnormalities of the eye (aniridia, Sturge-Weber syndrome, Peters anomaly, etc.), the eye's drainage pathways are not well developed, and this can cause glaucoma in children or secondary open-angle or angle-closure glaucoma in adults (see *Chapter 2*).

PROBABLE RISK FACTORS

Vascular risk factors

Several studies have shown that vascular risk factors (such as atherosclerosis, stroke, heart failure, angina, high cholesterol, high blood pressure and low blood pressure) can lead to primary open-angle glaucoma, mainly because of fluctuations in blood pressure. Fluctuations in ocular perfusion pressure (difference between arterial blood pressure and intraocular pressure) are also a possible cause. People with vasospasms (migraines, Raynaud's phenomenon, etc.) are also at higher risk of normal-tension glau-

WHAT DOES NOT CAUSE GLAUCOMA

There are quite a few common myths about glaucoma. Though we may not know exactly what causes glaucoma, we do know what does NOT cause it! Glaucoma is not caused by any of the following:

- Being a man or a woman (both men and women get glaucoma)
- Stress or anxiety
- Lack of sleep
- Poor diet
- Lack of vitamins
- Intensive use of the eyes (prolonged reading, working at a computer, etc.)
- Contact lenses
- Make-up
- Menopause
- Sexual activity
- Viagra
- Poor lighting
- Intense light
- Camera flashes

coma. A study published in 2006 reports cardiovascular disease in 17 percent of all patients with glaucoma.

Diabetes

People with diabetes appear to be at higher risk of developing secondary open-angle glaucoma. However, there is no consensus among specialists on recognition of diabetes as a risk factor. Some think glaucoma is detected more quickly in diabetics because of the eye problems associated with diabetes that require regular visits to the ophthalmologist. Until more in-depth studies of this risk factor have been conducted, diabetics are advised to have their intraocular pressure monitored.

Other diseases

Researchers have established links between secondary open-angle glaucoma and certain syndromes or diseases, such as hypothyroidism, sleep apnea and migraines. Further study is, however, required to confirm a definite a link between these disorders and glaucoma.

Smoking

Some studies show that smoking is a risk factor in open-angle glaucoma. We don't know exactly why, but we do know that smoking can cause vascular changes and thus damage the optic nerve. This may explain the link with glaucoma. Unlike age or family history, smoking is a risk factor over which the patient has some control. In other words, it is not only a probable risk factor but a modifiable risk factor as well.

ONE PERSON'S STORY

Name: Steven	**Age:** 49 years old

| **Occupation:** Electrician ||

Steven has known for a long time that he is at risk for glaucoma because his mother has been undergoing treatment for primary open-angle glaucoma for years and his maternal grandmother was blind when she died, probably because of glaucoma that was never diagnosed. Steven thus wants to maximize his chances of preserving his sight. He gets his intraocular pressure (IOP) checked by an optometrist annually, or at least every two years.

This year, the optometrist found Steven's intraocular pressure to be higher than in preceding years. Steven was not surprised, as he knows that age is a risk factor in glaucoma as well as family history. At 49, therefore, he now has an additional risk factor.

His optometrist referred him to an ophthalmologist, who noted his family history and checked not only his intraocular pressure but also the appearance of the optic nerve, the thickness of his cornea and his visual field. Though Steven's vision is not affected and he does not have glaucoma (there is no damage to his optic nerve), the ophthalmologist considers him a "glaucoma suspect," meaning that he is at risk of developing glaucoma. The ophthalmologist thus prescribed eye drops, to be applied daily in both eyes to reduce Steven's intraocular pressure and maintain it at a normal level. This will maximize Steven's chances of preventing his elevated intraocular pressure from progressing to glaucoma and damaging his vision.

CHAPTER 4
DIAGNOSIS

Glaucoma is diagnosed by looking for signs associated with the disease: elevated intraocular pressure, damage to the optic nerve and loss of peripheral vision. The goal of screening for glaucoma is to prevent vision loss through early detection (in a private clinic or hospital) and suitable intervention. Early diagnosis is especially important because glaucoma is a disease without symptoms in its early stages. A number of examinations are necessary to make a diagnosis. In case of doubt, the examinations are repeated every few months. If there is a change that suggests glaucoma, the diagnosis can be confirmed.

Based on results obtained with diagnostic devices, the ophthalmologist can determine not only the type of glaucoma but also the stage of the disease: early, moderate or advanced.

EARLY DETECTION

Early detection of glaucoma is crucial so that treatment and monitoring can begin as soon as possible. Treatments work better when the diagnosis is made early and they are administered in a timely fashion.

Everyone diagnosed with glaucoma must be followed regularly, the frequency of check-ups depending on the risks and the symptoms presented.

We cannot insist too much on the importance of routine eye examinations, even when vision seems normal, as glaucoma can remain asymptomatic for many years despite gradual deterioration of the optic nerve.

Of course, in case of one or more risk factors (see *Chapter 3*), screening is essential. Screening is strongly recommended for anyone over the age of 40 when one or more family members have glaucoma.

COMPREHENSIVE EYE EXAMINATION

In a comprehensive eye examination, a technician or vision specialist (optometrist or ophthalmologist) notes past health problems and performs certain tests. Most of the tests are performed at the first visit to establish a diagnosis but are not systematically performed at each follow-up visit. The ophthalmologist will decide which ones to repeat depending on the scope and speed of disease progression.

General health and eye health questionnaire

Before undertaking more specific examinations, the vision specialist will want to know about your general health (diabetes, hypertension, heart disease, allergies, etc.), your eye health (myopia, hypermetropia, surgery, etc.), your family history, age, ethnicity and any treatments or medication you are taking (to ensure they are not harmful to your eyes).

Visual acuity test

Vision is measured using a visual acuity chart called the Snellen chart or scale. The chart consists of rows of letters or drawings that decrease in size line by line. Vision specialists are referring to this chart when they speak of a gain or loss of a "line of visual acuity."

Visual acuity tests measure the sharpness of central vision, needed for seeing details clearly. Visual acuity scores are expressed as a fraction, not a percentage.

Normal vision is 6/6 (in metres) or 20/20 (in feet). The first number of the fraction represents the patient's distance from the Snellen chart. The second number shows the distance from which most people without a visual impairment would be able to read the line of letters on the chart (see box *Visual impairment*).

Though glaucoma can lead to blindness, most people with glaucoma have very good vision. It is only in the advanced stage of the disease, when the optic nerve is extensively damaged, that visual acuity diminishes. The ophthalmologist cannot base the diagnosis on a vision examination only.

Eye examination

An eye examination will show if you have other disorders that could cause an eventual loss of vision—such as age-related macular degeneration (AMD), cataracts or other eye diseases. The examin-

VISUAL IMPAIRMENT

Anyone whose visual acuity with an adequate optical correction is less than 6/21 (or 20/70) has a major visual impairment. This means the person can see at six metres (or 20 feet) an object that is generally perceived at 21 metres (or 70 feet) by someone with normal vision.

If central vision is 6/60 (20/200) or less, the person is considered legally blind.

ation includes an external examination of the eye and its adnexa (eyelids, tear glands and tear ducts), an evaluation of ocular motility (eye that deviates, excessive movement, etc.), a biomicroscopic (slit lamp) examination and intraocular pressure measurement.

WHEN SHOULD I SEE A DOCTOR?

Ophthalmological examinations are crucial, not only to diagnose glaucoma but also to track its development and assess the effect of treatment.

Examination frequency if you have symptoms
If you notice changes in visual acuity, visual field or colour vision, or physical changes to the eye, you should be examined as soon as possible.

Examination frequency if you are at high risk of developing glaucoma
If you are at risk of visual impairment (for example, if you have diabetes or cataracts or you are a glaucoma suspect), you should be examined more frequently and thoroughly:
Over 40 years of age: at least every three years
Over 50 years of age: at least every two years
Over 60 years of age: at least once a year

Examination frequency if you are without symptoms and at low risk
19 to 40 years of age: at least every 10 years
41 to 55 years of age: at least every five years
56 to 65 years of age: at least every three years
Over 65 years of age: at least every two years

Source: Canadian Ophthalmological Society clinical practice guidelines for periodic eye examination

Eye diseases other than glaucoma (cataracts, for example) can be detected with a biomicroscope examination, as can disorders that might explain elevated intraocular pressure and glaucoma—such as whitish or grey deposits on the lens (characteristic of pseudoexfoliative syndrome), abnormal blood vessels and pigment in the anterior chamber (typical of pigment dispersion syndrome). This information makes it possible to diagnose certain types of secondary glaucoma caused by eye disease (see *Chapter 3*).

Fundus examination

A fundus examination (examination of the back of the eye) is systematically performed at every check-up, as it allows the vision specialist to see the appearance, shape and colour of the optic disc (head of the optic nerve) and the retinal ganglion cells directly through the pupil. Thus any signs of damage to the optic nerve can be seen, a key element in diagnosing, staging and monitoring the progression of glaucoma and in verifying the effectiveness of treatments.

PUPIL DILATION

Pupil dilation is required for a proper fundus examination. However, in case of a narrow iridocorneal angle, the pupil is not dilated, as pupil dilation can increase angle closure. To dilate the pupil, drops are put in the eye that force the pupil to stay open. It takes about 15 minutes for the drops to take full effect. Pupil dilation is not painful, but the eyes may become sensitive to light and near vision can be disturbed for several hours. It is thus recommended that the patient bring a pair of sunglasses and either be accompanied or make arrangements for the trip home. Patients are advised not to drive for several hours after the examination.

To evaluate the quantity of nerve fibre that has not been affected by glaucoma, the ophthalmologist checks the size of the optic nerve cup (also called the optic disc cup), that is, the empty space created by the loss of optic nerve fibres. As the glaucoma progresses, the optic nerve fibres continue to die, and the cup becomes larger (see *Chapter 1*).

The doctor can also see if there is any hemorrhaging of the optic nerve for unknown reasons, another sign of glaucomatous damage.

A fundus examination can be performed in different ways: with an ophthalmoscope or a biomicroscope (slit lamp) (*Figure* ❶) and with or without a contact lens. Fundus photography can also be performed with a fundus camera during the examination to obtain images of the back of the eye (*Figure* ❷). Painless and harmless, a fundus examination often requires dilation of the pupil with drops (see box *Pupil dilation*) so the doctor can see more deeply into the eye, since the optic nerve is located at the back the eye. Ocular imaging examinations can provide more detailed information (see *Eye imaging* below in this chapter).

Measuring intraocular pressure (IOP)

Measurement of intraocular pressure is the basic test for diagnosing and monitoring glaucoma.

Intraocular pressure is measured by applying a tonometer to the eye with or without making contact with the cornea. The tonometer calculates intraocular pressure based on the force required to flatten the cornea by simple contact (Goldmann tonometer, Tono-Pen, Perkins tonometer, pneumotonometer, Pascal tonometer or Icare tonometer) or with a jet of air (air-puff tonometer or Ocular Response Analyser, ORA). The Goldmann tonometer is the device most commonly used. With this device, the eyes are first numbed with anesthetic drops, so the examination is painless. Next the cornea is gently pressed backward with a plastic applanation cone until an area of the cornea with a diameter of exactly 3.06 mm is flattened. The pressure applied to flatten this area of the cornea corresponds to the intraocular pressure. The flattening force

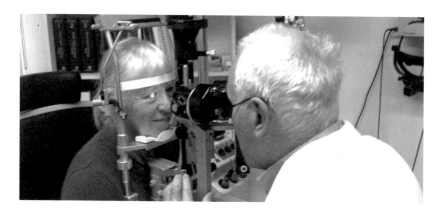

❶ Biomicroscope examination

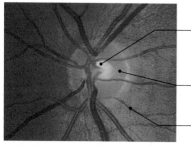

Optic nerve cupping or optic disc excavation (pale area)

Optic disc or optic nerve head (dark-coloured area)

Blood vessels

Normal optic disc

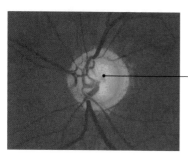

In this patient with glaucoma, the enlarged pale area (optic nerve cupping) indicates loss of retinal ganglion cells

Optic disc damaged by glaucoma

❷ Photos of the back of the eye

required is thus converted into millimetres of mercury (mm Hg) (*Figure* ❸).

Generally speaking, an exact measurement of intraocular pressure cannot be obtained. The result obtained is thus an estimate only, as the measurement can be biased by different factors, including the thickness of the cornea and fluctuations in intraocular pressure. Sometimes, a patient is kept under observation for an entire day so the doctor can check fluctuations in his or her intraocular pressure over an extended period of time.

The thickness of the cornea also has an impact on intraocular pressure measurements, as these are obtained by determining the force required to deform the eye—like pressing on a balloon to see if it is properly inflated. If the cornea is abnormally thick, however, it will flatten less easily, and intraocular pressure will be overestimated. On the other hand, if the cornea is abnormally thin, it will flatten more easily and intraocular pressure will be underestimated. The ophthalmologist will generally measure the thickness of your cornea (pachymetry) at your first visit, so the accuracy of subsequent intraocular pressure measurements can be understood. Corneal thickness can be measured with a number of devices. The most popular instrument for measuring corneal thickness, the ultrasound pachymeter, requires contact with the eye, which is first numbed with anesthetic drops. Optical coherence tomography (OCT), a Pentacam, an Orbiscan or corneal topography can be used to measure corneal thickness without contact with the eye. The examination is painless, lasts only a few seconds and does not need to be repeated at a later date, as corneal thickness does not change over time.

Iridocorneal angle examination (gonioscopy)

Iridocorneal angle examination (gonioscopy) is crucial in diagnosing open-angle or angle-closure glaucoma. Iridocorneal angle examinations are conducted periodically to check angle closure. The examination is painless, as anesthetic eye drops are first applied. At worst, the examination can cause mild discomfort. A cone-shaped contact lens (gonioscope) is placed on the cornea. The gonioscope

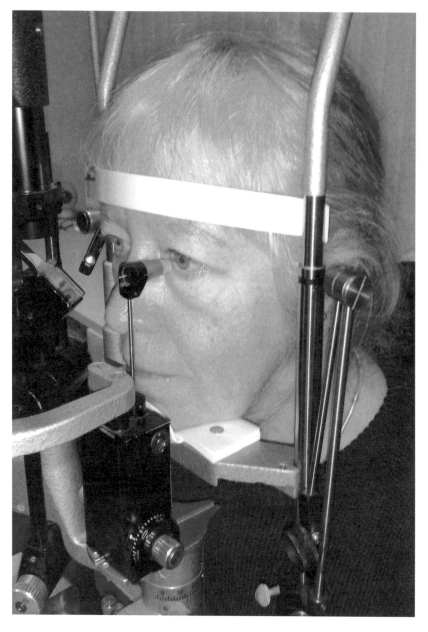

❸ Measuring intraocular pressure using a tonometer

contains mirrors placed at an angle so the ophthalmologist can use a biomicroscope (slit lamp) to examine the interior of the iridocorneal angle, which is otherwise inaccessible (*Figure* ❹).

Examination of the iridocorneal angle makes it possible, first of all, to detect anomalies in the trabecular meshwork that could hinder drainage of the aqueous humour (abnormal blood vessels, ruptures, pigment deposits, etc.). These anomalies are the cause of certain types of secondary open-angle glaucoma. Iridocorneal angle examination is also essential for diagnosing primary open-angle glaucoma, as it can eliminate angle-closure glaucoma or secondary open-angle glaucoma as a diagnosis.

Iridocorneal angle examination is also used to determine the degree of opening of the angle between the iris and the cornea, essential information in diagnosing and monitoring angle-closure glaucoma. The Shaffer grading system is used to assign a numerical grade to each angle based on anatomical description, angle width and implied clinical interpretation:

- Grade 4 (40°): widest angle, angle closure impossible
- Grade 3 (30°): open angle, angle closure impossible
- Grade 2 (20°): moderately narrow angle, only the trabecular meshwork can be identified, angle closure possible but unlikely, angle-closure glaucoma suspect
- Grade 1 (10°): very narrow angle, trabecular meshwork may be identifiable, angle closure not inevitable, but risk is high, angle-closure glaucoma suspect
- Grade 0 (0°): closed angle, no structures can be identified, angle-closure glaucoma

Iridocorneal angle examinations are performed regularly as part of the follow-up of patients who are angle-closure glaucoma suspects. Iridocorneal angle examinations may also be performed periodically in patients with open-angle glaucoma, as the iridocorneal angle is a dynamic structure that may evolve over time depending on the position of the lens or other factors. In other words, patients with primary open-angle glaucoma can, over the long term, present with angle-closure glaucoma as well.

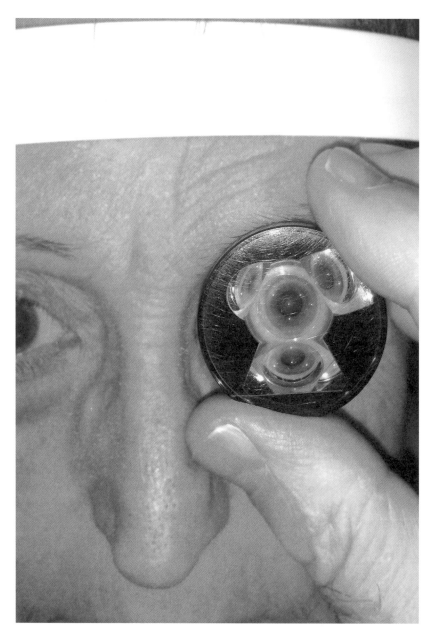

❹ Iridocorneal angle examination (gonioscopy)

Sometimes, eye imaging technologies, in particular OCT or UBM (see below in this chapter), are used to complete the angle examination.

Visual field test (perimetry test)

This examination is essential not only for diagnosing glaucoma but also for staging the disease (early, moderate or advanced). It is used to measure and map the scope of vision of each eye. The instrument used (a perimeter) detects even the smallest areas in your visual field where you see nothing or very little. Generally, we are not conscious of these "blank spots" in our vision, because the brain uses a variety of methods to fill them in and reconstruct an image that seems complete and coherent (*Figure* ❺).

This examination is completely painless. Each eye is tested separately for about three to six minutes with an automatic Humphrey or Octopus perimeter, an instrument with a bowl-shaped area into which you look. Random points of light will flash around different places in the bowl, and you will be asked to press a button whenever you see a light.

EYE IMAGING

Performed in a private clinic or a hospital, eye imaging is used to diagnose glaucoma and to monitor people with the disease. The technology or instrument used (OCT, HRT, GDx, UBM or photography) differs from one place to the next, but all make it possible to measure damage stemming from glaucoma. Data collected are compared to those in a normative database, allowing the doctor not only to determine the probability that the patient has glaucoma but also to stage the disease. Eye imaging is also performed at each check-up to track the progress of the disease. Further, eye imaging is very useful after eye surgery, to assess changes to the eyes.

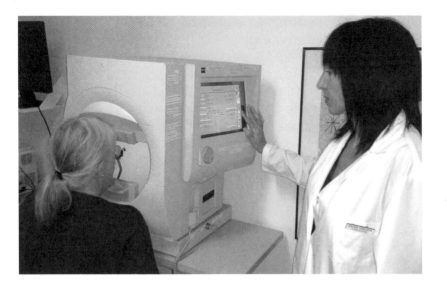

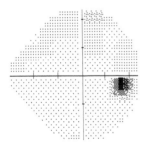

In a healthy eye, the areas of normal vision in the visual field appear lighter in the perimetry printout. The dark area indicates the normal blind spot that corresponds to the location of the optic nerve head, where there is no vision.

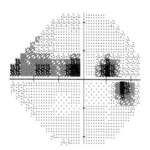

In this patient with glaucoma, damage to the optic nerve has caused a loss of vision in certain parts of the visual field. The spots (or darker areas) indicate damaged regions of the visual field. The black areas indicate places where there is no vision.

❺ Visual field test (perimetry test)

Optical coherence tomography (OCT)

Optical coherence tomography, or OCT, is like other types of medical scanning, except light is used instead of x-rays. The OCT scanner measures the time it takes for light (its speed) to travel through the ocular media and the retina before it is reflected back by tissues and structures. These measurements are used to generate very precise cross-sectional images of the eye's anterior segment (space between the cornea and the lens) and posterior segment (the ocular fundus).

The images of the anterior segment allow examination of the anatomical structures of the iridocorneal angle and provide information that cannot be obtained from an iridocorneal examination (see *Iridocorneal angle examination* above in this chapter). A light (slit lamp) is required to perform an iridocorneal angle examination (gonioscopy), but OCT can be performed in the dark. As light can alter the appearance of the angle by contracting the pupil and thus diminishing angle closure, the information obtained from OCT complements that obtained from iridocorneal angle examination (gonioscopy) and is essential in diagnosing certain forms of angle closure (such as plateau iris syndrome) and in assessing angle closure risk.

The images of the posterior segment of the eye allow examination of the optic disc, the retinal ganglion cells and the macula (*Figure* ❻). In particular, OCT can be used to measure cupping of the optic nerve head (optic disc), to quantify the remaining optic nerve fibers and to assess ganglion cell damage so a detailed diagnosis can be made.

The examination is not painful, as contact with the eye is not required. However, eye drops are often used to dilate the pupils so that better quality images can be obtained (see box *Pupil dilation*).

Other medical imaging technologies can be used to examine the optic disc and the retinal ganglion cells, including confocal scanning laser ophthalmoscopy (also called Heidelberg retina tomography or HRT) and scanning laser polarimetry (GDx).

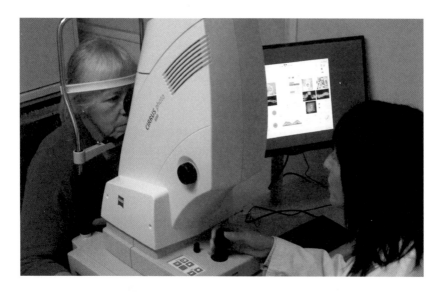

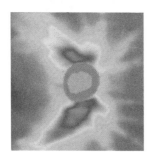

Normal OCT
Healthy eye with numerous retinal ganglion cells (red and yellow in the scan) penetrating the optic nerve (grey in the centre)

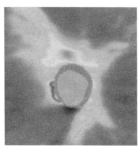

Abnormal OCT
In this patient with glaucoma, there is severe damage to the retinal ganglion cells, as indicated by the smaller amount of yellow and red, particularly in the lower part of the image.

❻ Optical coherence tomography (OCT) scanner

Ultrasound biomicroscopy (UBM)

Ultrasound biomicroscopy is a high-frequency ultrasound technology used to obtain information similar to that provided by OCT. Which technology is used to diagnose and monitor glaucoma depends on the equipment available at the clinic or hospital where the testing is performed.

Ultrasound biomicroscopy (UBM) makes it possible to obtain and analyze high-resolution videos and digital images of the different structures of the anterior segment of the eye (the cornea, iridocorneal angle, iris and lens) quickly and easily. In addition, it is easier to obtain images of the back of the iris with UBM than with OCT, facilitating detection of elements behind the iris (such as cysts or tumours) that can push the structures of the eye forward and cause the iridocorneal angle to close.

WHO DOES WHAT?

- **An optician** makes and sells corrective lenses according to a prescription written by an optometrist or an ophthalmologist. Opticians do not perform eye examinations.
- **Optometrists** are vision professionals but are not physicians. They are often the first practitioner consulted when vision problems arise. Based on a clinical eye examination, an optometrist can identify certain eye and vision problems, prescribe and/or sell glasses and, if need be, refer the patient to an ophthalmologist. In Quebec, an optometrist must refer the patient to a doctor (ophthalmologist or other physician) if he or she sees signs of disease. An optometrist may, however, treat certain minor ailments.
- **An ophthalmologist** is a medical doctor. He or she is trained to perform a complete assessment of visual function, make diagnoses and provide medical and surgical treatment of diseases or disorders of the eye and related structures (eyelids, tear glands, tear ducts and eyeball).

UBM is not painful, as contact with the eye is not required. In addition, pupil dilation is not necessary.

Fundus photography

Photography of the fundus or back of the eye is another technology used to observe the optic disc and the retinal ganglion cells (see *Figure* ❷ above in this chapter). However, this technology is becoming less and less popular, though it was the gold standard in diagnostic imaging for many years, and is gradually being replaced by OCT and HRT. Fundus photography is used to take photos of the optic nerve. The ophthalmologist then compares the photographs taken annually to check for changes in the structure of the optic nerve. This technology is less sensitive than the newer technologies in diagnosing or monitoring glaucoma. However, fundus photography makes it possible to see hemorrhages that cannot be seen with other technologies.

Fundus photography is not painful, as contact with the eye is not required. However, eye drops are used to dilate the pupils so that better quality images can be obtained (see box *Pupil dilation*).

ONE PERSON'S STORY

Name: Isabel	**Age:** 40 years old

Occupation: Musician

Isabel has been myopic since she was a child and is followed regularly by an optometrist. During her last eye examination, her optometrist found that her intraocular pressure (IOP) was higher than average, at 23 mm Hg, and referred her to an ophthalmologist. The ophthalmologist also found that her intraocular pressure was elevated and proceeded to perform other examinations to determine the cause of the elevated pressure. A visual acuity test and a visual field examination did not show any vision impairment. Corneal thickness measurement (using an ultrasound pachymeter), however, yielded elevated results. Isabel's thick cornea was thus probably the reason for the elevated intraocular pressure measurement. A gonioscopic examination of the iridocorneal angle proved normal. To make sure Isabel did not have glaucoma, the ophthalmologist used an ophthalmoscope to examine her optic nerves and then confirmed the observations made in the ophthalmoscopic examinations with optical coherence tomography (OCT). Finding nothing abnormal, the ophthalmologist concluded that Isabel does not have glaucoma. He explained to her that there was no cause for concern, that the elevated intraocular pressure was related to her cornea, which was thicker than usual. Isabel was referred once again to her optometrist, who would be responsible not only for regular follow-up on her myopia but also for checking that her intraocular pressure did not increase in the future. This follow-up is especially important, as myopia is a risk factor in primary open-angle glaucoma and pigmentary glaucoma.

CHAPTER 5
PREVENTION
AND TREATMENT

Glaucoma cannot be cured, but it can be treated. This means that damage already done is irreversible but the disease can be controlled to prevent loss of vision. The main objective of treatment is to lower intraocular pressure. With each patient, the ophthalmologist determines the target intraocular pressure based on a number of elements, in particular intraocular pressure before starting treatment, the stage of the disease and the visual field damage.

Three types of therapy are used: drug therapy, laser treatments and surgery. Treatment is selected depending on the type and stage of the glaucoma. The different types of open-angle and angle-closure glaucoma do not all require the same treatment. Treatments may also be combined in certain cases.

We also know that angle-closure glaucoma can turn into open-angle glaucoma when elevated intraocular pressure persists after laser therapy. In other words, the treatment required can change over the course of the disease.

Fortunately, existing treatments make it possible to live a completely normal life with glaucoma because they prevent major vision loss. However, prevention depends on real collaboration of the person who has the disease.

PREVENTING GLAUCOMA OR ITS PROGRESSION

There is currently no way to prevent the onset of glaucoma—with the exception of acute angle-closure glaucoma attack, which may be prevented by an iridotomy (see *Iridotomy* below in this chapter). However, it is possible with all other types of glaucoma, once diagnosed, to maximize the chances of preventing progression of the disease and maintaining good eyesight. The best way to do this is to follow the treatment recommended by your doctor, without fail. Unless your doctor recommends otherwise, it is dangerous to stop using eye drops for any extended period of time. If treatment is discontinued, intraocular pressure rises and vision will gradually deteriorate. It is thus important to inform your attending medical team of

DENIAL OF THE DISEASE

Denial (categorical refusal to acknowledge the disease) is not uncommon in people with glaucoma. It can be straightforward, with an outright refusal of care. It can also be unconscious, taking the form of failure to take prescribed medication or have regular eye examinations. Some deny the disease because they feel that accepting it will mean restrictions. Others feel they are invincible. Still others don't understand the importance of following their doctor's recommendations, especially when they don't have any symptoms. It is thus crucial to remind those with glaucoma of the importance of regular monitoring.

any side effects so that another medical or surgical solution can be considered to reduce intraocular pressure.

Remember as well that glaucoma can remain asymptomatic until it reaches an advanced stage. Regular eye examinations are thus vital, particularly if you have one or more risk factors (see *Chapter 3*), such as a family history of glaucoma.

DRUG THERAPIES

Existing drugs target the main risk factor in open-angle as well as angle-closure glaucoma: elevated intraocular pressure. The goal is to achieve and maintain a target intraocular pressure below the pressure at which optic nerve fibre loss is observed. This target intraocular pressure varies from one person to the next. There is no magic number that will systematically lead to stabilization of the disease.

Most drug therapies for glaucoma are prescribed for life, and it is important that they never be discontinued (barring contraindications or adverse effects). Otherwise, the disease may progress and cause narrowing of the visual field and eventually blindness. On your doctor's recommendation, however, drug therapies can be reduced or discontinued after laser treatment or surgery (see below in this chapter), if the procedure leads to a sufficient lowering of intraocular pressure. Drug therapies may also be prescribed after laser therapy or surgery if the procedure does not lead to a satisfactory lowering of intraocular pressure.

Most existing drug therapies come in the form of drops that are placed in one or both eyes. Antiangiogenics are the exception, as they are administered by injection.

Drug therapies reduce intraocular pressure using different mechanisms of action: some diminish the production of aqueous humour in the eye while others facilitate its drainage.

The ophthalmologist decides which treatment is best based on signs and symptoms presented and the progression of the disease. He or she may also modify the treatment or prescribe additional therapy if the prescribed treatment proves less effective over time, the glaucoma progresses or side effects appear.

Prostaglandin analogues

Prostaglandin analogues are the newest eye drops for the treatment of glaucoma. They first appeared on the market in 1996 and are currently the eye drops most frequently prescribed for glaucoma. They lower intraocular pressure by increasing aqueous humour outflow through the uveoscleral pathway (see *The trabecular meshwork and the uveoscleral pathway* in *Chapter 1*).

The recommended dose is one drop per day in the affected eye, preferably in the evening, as the drops tend to cause the eyes to get red. Prostaglandin analogues must not be used more than once a day. If you forget to apply the drops, it is best to wait till the following day and apply them at the usual time. Never double the dose to compensate for a missed dose. An overdose can have the opposite effect to that desired, that is, it can increase intraocular pressure instead of lowering it. Though it is recommended that the drops be applied every day at the same time, a little leeway is allowed on the timing.

Unopened bottles of prostaglandin analogues containing latanoprost should be kept in the refrigerator. Once opened, they can be kept at room temperature. Other prostaglandin analogues do not need to be refrigerated.

Side effects

Prostaglandin analogues can cause darkening of the colour of the iris, particularly in people with hazel eyes. These eye drops can also cause an increase in thickness, length and quantity of eyelashes. Also, fine hair sometimes starts to grow under the eyelid. In addition, the treatment can change the color of the skin around the eyes, reduce orbital fat (fat surrounding the eye) and cause conjunctival redness and a burning sensation inside the eye when applied. Prostaglandin analogues have few known systemic adverse effects (that is, they do not affect other organs in the body).

Beta blockers

Beta blockers have been available since 1978. Though they have few ocular side effects, they are not used as frequently as prostaglandin analogues because they may be less effective in lowering

---

HOW TO PUT IN YOUR EYE DROPS

First, wash your hands thoroughly and remove your contact lenses, if you are wearing any. You can lie down to apply the drops, or just tilt your head slightly backwards. Next, look up and gently pull your lower lid down. With your other hand, bring the eye dropper as close as you can to your eye without touching it, and squeeze one drop into the pocket formed in your lower lid. To make sure that the drop actually went in your eye, you can keep the eye drop bottle in the refrigerator, as it is easier to feel a cold drop than a drop at room temperature. Close your eyes after applying the drop and keep them closed for several minutes, so the drop will stay in contact with your eye as long as possible rather than running into the tear duct or your nostrils. You can also press with your finger between your eye and your nose to close off the tear drainage duct. This will prevent the drug from getting into the bloodstream and reduce side effects that certain drops can have on other organs. If you wear contact lenses, there are a number of specific recommendations (see box *Contact lenses* in *Chapter 6*).

Make sure you always have a new bottle of eye drops on hand so you won't ever have to stop your treatment. In addition, check with your pharmacist to make sure your prescription is renewable. If necessary, call your ophthalmologist and ask for a renewal until your next appointment. If your ophthalmologist is unavailable, your family doctor can renew the prescription for your drops for a month until your ophthalmologist returns.

intraocular pressure. Beta blockers are prescribed mainly when the patient cannot tolerate prostaglandin analogues, when glaucoma is found in one eye only or when prostaglandin analogues are unable to adequately control intraocular pressure. They are also used to reduce intraocular pressure after eye surgery, as prostaglandin analogues tend to aggravate inflammation caused by surgery. For the same reason, beta blockers are also preferred for lowering intraocular pressure in patients with chronic inflammatory eye disorders.

Beta blocker eye drops lower intraocular pressure by reducing the secretion of aqueous humour. To do so, the drug inhibits the action of the sympathetic nervous system (one of the two parts of the autonomous nervous system), which is involved in the production of aqueous humour.

As activation of the sympathetic nervous system takes place when we are awake, beta blocker eye drops are applied in the morning.

The dose is one drop in each eye once or twice a day, as prescribed by your doctor.

Side effects

Beta blockers have few adverse effects on the eyes, apart from dryness. However, they are contraindicated (not advised) in people with asthma, emphysema, bradycardia, chronic obstructive pulmonary disease (COPD) and certain heart problems because they might get into the bloodstream. Beta blockers can also mask certain signs of hypoglycemia (heart palpitations) in people with diabetes, and they can cause a drop in blood pressure. Patients have reported problems with sexual dysfunction and depression; however, studies have not confirmed any association with beta blockers, and these adverse effects could be related to receiving a diagnosis of glaucoma.

Carbonic anhydrase inhibitors

Carbonic anhydrase inhibitors have been available in oral form (tablets) since 1954 and in topical form (drops) since 1991. They can also be given as an intravenous infusion, in particular to treat the rare cases of acute angle-closure glaucoma attack.

Though the tablets are more effective than the drops, they are not often used as they can have major side effects.

Carbonic anhydrase inhibitors may be prescribed for several weeks before a surgical procedure if the surgery cannot be performed rapidly and intraocular pressure remains too high despite administration of other medicines. The ophthalmologist will then add carbonic anhydrase inhibitors to the other drops.

Carbonic anhydrase inhibitors act on intraocular pressure by suppressing the secretion of aqueous humour.

Carbonic anhydrase inhibitor drops are applied two to three times a day. Tablets are taken two to four times a day.

Side effects
In the form of eye drops, carbonic anhydrase inhibitors can cause an allergic reaction that manifests as stinging of the eyes on application of the drops, itchy, red eyes and sometimes swelling of the cornea.

In tablet form, carbonic anhydrase inhibitors can cause a number of adverse effects, including changes in the taste of food, tingling in the hands and feet, nausea, diarrhea, loss of appetite, fatigue, dizziness, insomnia, an increase in frequency of urination, depression, kidney stones, anemia and skin allergies. They may also cause myopia, acute angle-closure glaucoma attack and choroidal detachment.

Alpha agonists
First marketed in 1988, alpha agonists are a little less effective than prostaglandin analogues but as effective as beta blockers in reducing intraocular pressure in people with glaucoma. However, they can trigger eyelid inflammation and allergic conjunctivitis in the medium term. They are often prescribed on a short-term basis after laser therapy to minimize the sudden increases in intraocular pressure that often occur after such procedures.

WHAT IF I AM PREGNANT OR BREASTFEEDING?

Any drug taken by mouth or in the form of a tablet will go into your bloodstream. This means that if you are pregnant or breastfeeding, the active ingredient could be transmitted to your unborn child or end up in your breast milk. The possible risks of glaucoma drug therapies to the unborn child or nursing infant of a woman with glaucoma are, however, poorly documented, controversial or simply unknown. It is thus recommended that women with glaucoma who are or plan to become pregnant inform their ophthalmologist as quickly as possible to discuss treatment options. The ophthalmologist will assess the risks and benefits of the treatment for the mother and the unborn child. Some of the following measures can be taken, depending on the stage of the glaucoma:

- The treatment can be discontinued for the first weeks of the pregnancy (the period during which the baby's main organs are formed) if intraocular pressure is not so elevated as to place the mother's optic nerve at risk.
- When treatment is essential, certain measures must be taken to minimize passage of the drug into the blood stream of the pregnant woman or the breast milk of the nursing mother. Studies show that this passage can be largely reduced by keeping the eyes closed (without blinking) after instilling the drops and putting manual pressure on the tear drainage duct, at the inside corner of the eye, for about five minutes.
- If you are breastfeeding, your ophthalmologist will discuss your treatment options with you based on your priorities. Though relatively little of the active ingredients in eye drops or tablets passes into breast milk, it is nonetheless possible to reduce this amount by taking the drug immediately after nursing, as this will minimize concentrations of the active ingredient in the breast milk at the next feeding. Of course, feeding the baby humanized milk instead, at least temporarily, is always an option.

Alpha agonist drops act in two ways: they suppress secretion of aqueous humour and they slightly increase its outflow. They do this by stimulating parts of the sympathetic nervous system.

Alpha agonist drops are applied in the eye affected by glaucoma two to three times a day, as recommended by your doctor.

Side effects

A common side effect of alpha agonist drops is eye allergy symptoms. As many as 40 percent of users of alpha agonist drops experience such symptoms: eye redness, stinging and irritation, and eyelid edema (swelling). Other adverse effects include nose and mouth dryness, fatigue, headache and fluctuations in blood pressure.

Cholinergics (or parasympathomimetics)

Cholinergics are our oldest glaucoma medication, in use since 1896.

Cholinergic drops are less frequently used today, as they cause adverse effects in the eyes. However, they are very often used in angle-closure glaucoma in patients who are aphakic (absent eye lens) or pseudophakic (natural eye lens has been replaced by an intraocular lens).

Cholinergics lower intraocular pressure by improving aqueous humour outflow. They cause the muscles of the ciliary body to contract, opening the trabecular meshwork.

Cholinergic drops are applied in the eye two to four times a day.

Side effects

Cholinergic drugs often cause adverse effects in the eyes, including constriction of the pupil (difficulty seeing in the dark) and increased myopia. At any rate, cholinergic drops must be used with caution in people with myopia, as they can cause retinal tearing and detachment.

Combination drops

It is not unusual for an ophthalmologist to prescribe two or more different kinds of eye drops for a patient to further reduce intraocular pressure. The different drops should be applied at least five minutes apart, but in no particular order. However, to reduce the number of drops that must be applied every day and prevent confusion between eye drop bottles, it is now possible to obtain two different drugs in one bottle (a beta blocker and a prostaglandin analogue, for example).

Adverse effects of the combination drops are the same as those when the drugs are each in a separate bottle, but any side effects from preservative agents will be reduced as they are only needed in one bottle. In addition, combination drops make it easier to administer the treatment and improve treatment compliance.

Antiangiogenics

Researchers made a major breakthrough in late 2004 with the use of antiangiogenics, or antivascular endothelial growth factor (anti-VEGF) agents, in the treatment of a number of eye diseases, including neovascular glaucoma (see *Chapter 2*). These drugs neutralize the activity of vascular endothelial growth factor (VEGF), which triggers growth of the new abnormal blood vessels characteristic of neovascular glaucoma. Injected directly into the eyes, antiangiogenics block development of these abnormal blood vessels in the iridocorneal angle, and in some cases this lowers intraocular pressure. Laser treatments (laser retinal photocoagulation) are then performed to destroy the cells that produce the vascular growth factor. Generally, the injections are discontinued after the laser treatment.

Two antiangiogenic agents are currently available in Canada, ranibizumab (Lucentis®) and bevacizumab (Avastin®), but only ranibizumab is recognized by Health Canada for ophthalmological use.

How is the treatment given?

The treatment is given in your doctor's office or a hospital under local anesthesia. The antiangiogenic agent is injected into the white of the eye. This only takes a few seconds. The procedure is not painful and is well tolerated by patients.

The therapy generally consists of a series of monthly injections, the exact number depending on the abnormal vessel growth observed by the ophthalmologist in the iridocorneal angle examination.

Side effects

Complications stemming from injections to the eye are very rare. It is normal for the eye to be mildly irritated following the treatment. Elevation of intraocular pressure is also possible. In one out of 1,000 injections, infection occurs inside the eyeball (endophthalmitis), in which case the eye becomes red and very painful, there is significant vision loss and an emergency trip to the hospital is required.

LASER TREATMENTS

Lasers are devices that generate a very precise beam of concentrated light energy. Laser beams can cut or burn living tissue to which they are applied. One of the advantages of laser treatments for eye problems is that they are painless and well tolerated. They are also performed very quickly and do not require hospitalization.

In people with glaucoma, lasers are used to reduce intraocular pressure and to treat certain forms of angle-closure glaucoma. In open-angle glaucoma, laser treatments are generally second-line therapy, used when eye drops do not sufficiently reduce intraocular pressure or when drops or tablets are not well tolerated. However, laser trabeculoplasty is becoming more and more common as first-line therapy, as it means people with glaucoma do not have to apply eye drops on a daily basis. Laser treatments are also considered as an option when surgery is risky—in elderly people with heart problems, for example.

Trabeculoplasty

To perform a trabeculoplasty, a laser beam is directed at the trabecular meshwork, causing the tissue to shrink and improving drainage of aqueous fluid out of the eye (*Figure* ❶). The laser treatment also helps the immune system get rid of waste in the trabecular meshwork and stimulates the creation of new cells.

Argon laser trabeculoplasty, the standard treatment for many years, is gradually being replaced by selective laser trabeculoplasty (SLT). The only difference between the two procedures is the type of laser used. SLT is a relatively new procedure (2001) that is performed with a frequency-doubled laser which emits a low-intensity beam that can target only the cells that react to the laser without affecting the rest of the trabecular meshwork. Instead of causing burns on the trabecular meshwork, a selective laser trabeculoplasty causes small localized reactions, which means more than two treatments over the course of a lifetime are possible.

Trabeculoplasty can be used to treat primary open-angle glaucoma, corticosteroid-induced secondary glaucoma, pigmentary glaucoma, exfoliative glaucoma or angle-closure glaucoma when an iridotomy is not successful in normalizing intraocular pressure (see *Iridotomy* below in this chapter).

The treatment can be as effective in lowering intraocular pressure as prostaglandins. The drop in pressure normally occurs several days after the procedure but can sometimes take several weeks. If intraocular pressure is still too high after the procedure, your doctor will prescribe eye drops for daily application. The effect of a trabeculoplasty can disappear with time, so the procedure may have to be performed a second or even a third time. However, the risks of side effects are greater when the procedure is repeated and the treatment may also be less effective.

How is the treatment given?

Trabeculoplasty is painless and may be performed in a hospital or in your ophthalmologist's office. It is generally performed in two sessions several weeks apart, one eye at a time or both eyes together. A drop of an alpha agonist is applied before or after the treatment to make sure that intraocular pressure does not increase too much after the procedure due to inflammation. Eye drops are

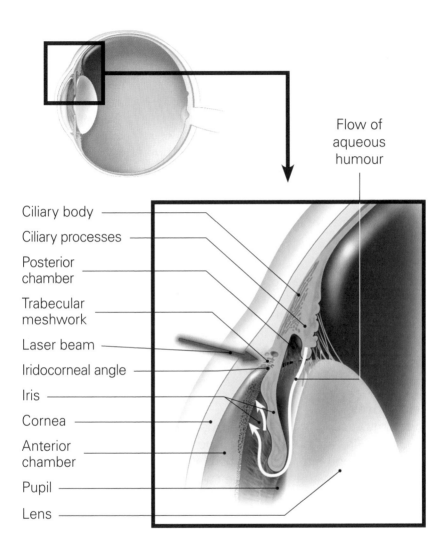

Ciliary body

Ciliary processes

Posterior chamber

Trabecular meshwork

Laser beam

Iridocorneal angle

Iris

Cornea

Anterior chamber

Pupil

Lens

Flow of aqueous humour

In a trabeculoplasty, a laser beam (red arrow) is directed at the trabecular meshwork. The beam cleans up the trabecular meshwork, increasing its capacity to drain the aqueous humour and thus leading to a drop in intraocular pressure.

❶ Trabeculoplasty

used to numb your eye. The ophthalmologist then places a magnifying contact lens on the cornea so the trabecular meshwork can be clearly seen, and a circular laser beam is directed onto the trabecular meshwork for several minutes. Some patients feel a slight sensation in the eye when the laser is applied.

After the laser therapy, you may have blurry vision because of the gel used to make the contact lens adhere to the eye during the procedure, but your vision will return to normal within minutes. This means that you don't necessarily need someone to drive you home after the procedure.

Anti-inflammatory drops may be prescribed for several days to prevent inflammation.

Side effects

In most cases, the procedure does not cause serious side effects and you can return to work and your usual activities on the following day. Sometimes the treatment causes a temporary increase in intraocular pressure in the hours following the procedure despite all the precautions taken to prevent this. Uveitis or changes to the cornea (hypermetropia) may occur, but this is rare.

Iridotomy

Iridotomy is used to treat angle-closure glaucoma. In this type of glaucoma, the aqueous humour is no longer able to flow between the anterior and the posterior chambers of the eye because of an obstruction between the iris (the coloured part of the eye) and the lens. As a result, aqueous humour collects in the posterior chamber, pushing on the iris and causing it to bulge forward and sometimes to obstruct the trabecular meshwork. An iridotomy involves using a laser to make a small hole in the iris that allows fluid to flow into the anterior chamber. The iris thus falls back into its normal position, opening the iridocorneal angle and allowing the aqueous humour to circulate normally once again (*Figure* ❷). The size of the hole created in the iris is variable and is determined by your ophthalmologist, but it is always too small to be seen by the naked eye.

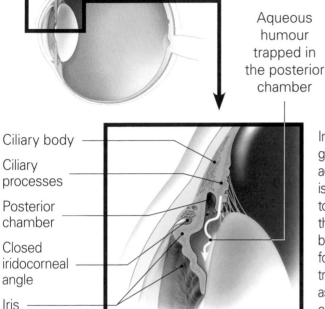

Aqueous humour trapped in the posterior chamber

Ciliary body

Ciliary processes

Posterior chamber

Closed iridocorneal angle

Iris

In angle-closure glaucoma, the aqueous humour is no longer able to circulate towards the anterior chamber. The iris is forced into the trabecular meshwork as a result and obstructs it.

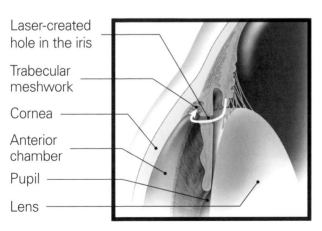

Laser-created hole in the iris

Trabecular meshwork

Cornea

Anterior chamber

Pupil

Lens

An iridotomy involves making a hole in the iris between the posterior and the anterior chambers and thus restoring normal flow of the aqueous humour.

❷ Iridotomy

Iridotomy is used mainly to treat acute angle-closure glaucoma attack or to prevent complete closure of the iridocorneal angle in susceptible patients.

In most cases, the procedure is successful in opening the iridocorneal angle. If the iridocorneal angle remains narrow after an iridotomy, other procedures must be considered, such as a peripheral iridoplasty (see *Peripheral iridoplasty* below in this chapter).

The hole created in the iris may remain permeable for life, but it may also close up with time, especially if there are cysts that push on it. Iridotomy can be repeated, but this is very rare.

How is the treatment given?

Iridotomies are performed in a hospital or in an ophthalmologist's office under local anesthesia (numbing eye drops). Both eyes can be treated on the same day or in two sessions. The procedure is painless and takes less than five minutes per eye.

A contact lens is placed on the eye to keep it open, provide a magnified view of the area to be treated and focus the laser light on the iris. Once the laser is focused on the target, a few brief laser pulses are delivered to pierce a small opening in the iris. You may hear a clicking sound and feel a pinch-like sensation. Your vision may be temporarily reduced after the treatment, mainly due to the gel used to make the contact lens stick to the eye and the dispersal of pigment caused by the procedure. Pigment dispersion can also cause intraocular pressure to rise. As it takes several hours for vision and intraocular pressure to return to normal, you may not drive after the procedure.

Side effects

In most cases, an iridotomy does not have any serious side effects and you can return to work and your usual activities the following day. The procedure can sometimes cause bleeding of the iris and slight swelling of the eye, but these complications can be easily treated by applying eye drops for several days and will not affect your vision.

Sometimes the opening made in the iris allows more light to pass through than usual, in which case you will see thin slightly discoloured horizontal lines in your vision that seem to move. Though this visual disorder is permanent, it is not serious and tends to become less bothersome with time.

Other complications can occur, such as corneal or lens damage, but they are rare. In addition, occasionally the hole created in the iris will close up.

Peripheral iridoplasty

Peripheral iridoplasty consists in applying a series of argon laser pulses to the peripheral iris tissue to thin it out. This procedure is mainly used in cases of primary angle-closure glaucoma with plateau iris syndrome (see *Chapter 2*). With this type of glaucoma, thinning of the iris reopens the iridocorneal angle, allowing the aqueous humour to drain.

How is the treatment given?

The procedure is the same as for an iridotomy (see *Iridotomy* above in this chapter).

Side effects

Possible side effects are the same as those observed after an iridotomy (see *Iridotomy* above in this chapter).

Laser cyclophotocoagulation

This laser therapy consists in destroying part of the ciliary body (eye tissue that produces the aqueous humour) by applying a laser beam to the sclera (outer envelope of the eye). Sometimes fibre optics are used and the laser beam is applied to the ciliary body itself (endocyclophotocoagulation, ECP). The procedure reduces aqueous humour secretion, which leads to a drop in intraocular pressure.

This procedure is generally used in glaucoma only when the risk of blindness is very high, when other treatments to lower intraocular pressure cannot be used or have proved unsuccessful, or when other surgical options have been exhausted. As endocyclophotocoagulation (ECP) is less invasive, it is sometimes used in combination with cataract surgery.

Intraocular pressure drops in the days following the procedure, but it is not uncommon for it to climb back up several years or even several months later. The treatment can then be repeated.

How is the treatment given?

Laser cyclophotocoagulation is usually painless. It is performed in a hospital or your ophthalmologist's office under local anesthesia (injection behind the eye, through the eyelid). It takes about ten minutes to do.

Side effects

Laser cyclophotocoagulation can cause inflammation of the eyes. This can be treated by taking anti-inflammatories for several days. Other adverse effects include discomfort, eye pain, eye hemorrhaging, eye redness lasting several weeks and temporary vision impairment due to macular edema (swelling of the macula) which becomes permanent in some cases (5 to 10 percent).

SURGERY

Surgery is used to treat all types of glaucoma and is often considered when other options (drug therapies and laser treatments) are unsuccessful in lowering intraocular pressure and controlling the progression of glaucoma. Surgery is used to restore the natural drainage pathway of the aqueous humour or to create a new drainage pathway. In either case, the goal is to lower intraocular pressure. Which type of surgery will be performed depends on the type of glaucoma you have, your ophthalmologist's opinion and the technologies available in the institution where the procedure will be performed. In some cases, your doctor may recommend a second surgery.

Trabeculectomy

Trabeculectomy is one of the oldest surgical interventions used to treat glaucoma (*Figure* ❸). It is a microsurgical procedure that consists in creating a new aqueous humour outflow system because aqueous humour drainage via the natural pathways is inadequate (see *The trabecular meshwork and the uveoscleral pathway* in *Chapter 1*).

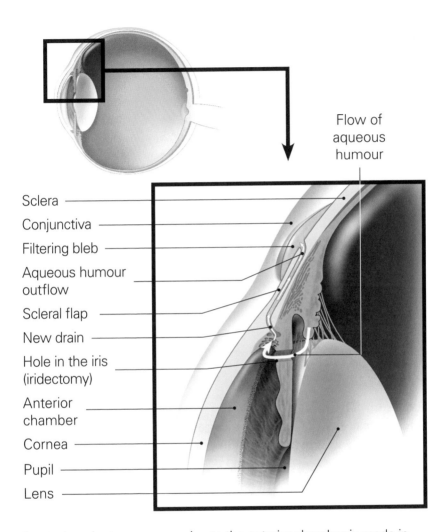

Flow of aqueous humour

Sclera

Conjunctiva

Filtering bleb

Aqueous humour outflow

Scleral flap

New drain

Hole in the iris (iridectomy)

Anterior chamber

Cornea

Pupil

Lens

In a trabeculectomy, an opening to the anterior chamber is made in the sclera (scleral flap). This allows the aqueous humour to drain out of the eye, bypassing the damaged trabecular meshwork. The aqueous humour accumulates under the conjunctiva, forms a little blister or bubble (called a "filtering bleb") and is eventually resorbed into the bloodstream or drains through the conjunctiva.

❸ Trabeculectomy

The first step in creating the new drainage system is to make a flap in the sclera. This scleral flap is essentially a small trap door that the ophthalmologist creates by cutting a flap half the thickness of the sclera through which the aqueous humour can drain out of the eye. A small hole into the anterior chamber of the eye is made under the scleral flap by removing part of the cornea and the trabecular meshwork. The scleral flap is sutured back in place with several stitches to control the rate of outflow of the aqueous humour. The ophthalmologist can adjust the rate of outflow even after the surgery by removing some of the stitches with a laser.

The trabeculectomy causes formation of a filtering bleb (see box *Post-operative filtering blebs*) underneath the conjunctiva through which aqueous humour can drain, causing intraocular pressure to drop. To prevent the iris from plugging the hole of the trabeculectomy and blocking aqueous humour outflow, an iridectomy (hole in the iris) is often performed as well. A possible complication in the short or long term is scarring of the conjunctiva or under the sclera flap, which can cause a rise in intraocular pressure several weeks, months or years later. Antimetabolites are often used during the surgery to reduce scarring.

ExPress Shunt

An ExPress Shunt is a drainage implant used to create a new outflow pathway for the aqueous humour. Instead of removing part of the trabecular meshwork and the cornea, as in a trabeculectomy, a tube is installed under the scleral flap created by the ophthalmologist (small trap door made in the sclera [see *Trabeculectomy* above in this chapter]) and inserted in the anterior chamber (*Figure* ❹). This means an iridectomy (hole in the iris) is not required. A number of studies have demonstrated that there are fewer risks of complications with this technology—less chance of choroid detachment or anterior chamber collapse—than with a trabeculectomy. However, this procedure is not performed in all hospitals because of the cost and the possible long-term complications, which are still poorly understood. As with a trabeculectomy, this procedure generally causes formation of a filtering bleb.

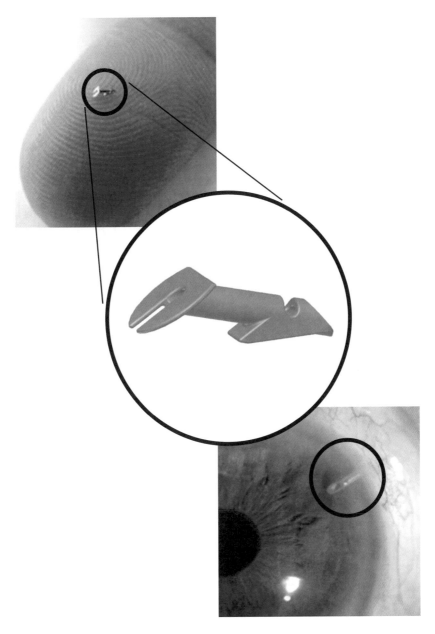

❹ ExPress Shunt

Glaucoma drainage implant

These implants create a new outflow channel for the aqueous humour in the posterior part of the eye. Surgery is required to insert them in your eyes. Often the ophthalmologist will opt for a drainage implant only after a trabeculectomy or an ExPress shunt has failed to achieve the desired results. There are several models available, including the Molteno, Ahmed and Baerveldt drainage implants. The implant consists of a small silicone tube that is inserted in the anterior chamber of the eye and connected to a silicone or plastic plate that is attached to the sclera (*Figure* ❺). The device promotes aqueous humour flow to neighbouring tissue, reducing intraocular pressure.

A donor tissue graft is often used to cover the tube and prevent the implant from moving out of place. Regular check-ups by an ophthalmologist are essential if you have this procedure to make sure you are not experiencing adverse effects.

TYPE OF SURGERY DEPENDS ON TYPE OF GLAUCOMA

The type of surgery selected for you depends on the type of glaucoma you have:

- Primary open-angle glaucoma: trabeculectomy, ExPress Shunt, glaucoma drainage implant, non-penetrating deep sclerectomy (NPDS), canaloplasty, trabectome surgery, trabecular bypass stent (iStent), suprachoroidal implant (gold micro shunt), cataract surgery (lens extraction).
- Angle-closure glaucoma: trabeculectomy, ExPress Shunt, glaucoma drainage implant, cataract surgery (lens extraction), vitrectomy.

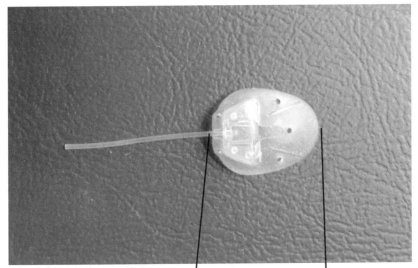

Ahmed drainage implant

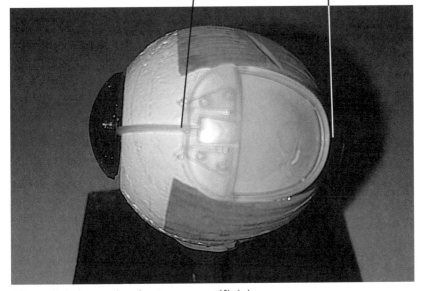

Ahmed drainage implant on an artificial eye

❺ Ahmed drainage implant

Non-penetrating deep sclerectomy (NPDS)

Non-penetrating deep sclerectomy (NPDS) is a variant of trabeculectomy. Instead of removing the cornea and the trabecular meshwork down to the anterior chamber, the surgeon leaves a thin layer of the cornea and the trabecular meshwork. The aqueous humour is then able to escape through this thin layer, like coffee percolating through a filter. Some surgeons insert a collagen micro-implant under the scleral flap they have created to prevent scarring of the tissue. The advantage of this procedure is that drops in pressure and intraocular bleeding are less common than with a trabeculectomy. The filtering blebs also tend to be smaller than with a trabeculectomy, reducing the risk of infection over the long term. The drawback is that NPDS sometimes does not lower intraocular pressure as much as a trabeculectomy.

Canaloplasty

Canaloplasty is always preceded by a non-penetrating deep sclerectomy (NPDS), as this gives the ophthalmologist access to the canal of Schlemm (see *Chapter 1*), a vein-like structure behind the trabecular meshwork through which the aqueous humour is drained. The ophthalmologist threads a suture through the canal of Schlemm (which runs 360 degrees internally inside the eye) and then tightens it slightly to create some tension before tying it. The tension helps the canal stay open, allowing the aqueous humour to drain through its natural outflow path. This procedure lowers intraocular pressure without removing part of the cornea and the trabecular meshwork and making a hole in the anterior chamber (as in a trabeculectomy). In addition, in many cases a filtering bleb is not created. However, sometimes the canal of Schlemm drainage system does not resume its natural function and other measures are required to lower intraocular pressure.

Trabectome surgery

This surgical procedure involves removing the strip of trabecular meshwork between the anterior chamber and the canal of Schlemm, which, according to a number of studies, is the tissue causing major resistance to aqueous humour outflow in open-angle glaucoma. This procedure re-establishes access to the aqueous humour's natural drainage pathway.

The surgery is performed with an electrocautery device that cuts, irrigates and aspirates tissue, cauterizing (purifying) it at the same time.

Cortisone drops are prescribed after the procedure to reduce scarring. The doctor must examine the iridocorneal angle regularly to make sure that the opening created is not closed over by scarring.

POST-OPERATIVE FILTERING BLEBS

After a trabeculectomy (see *Trabeculectomy* above in this chapter), a little blister or bubble, called a "filtering bleb," generally forms on the conjunctiva, hidden under the upper eyelid. The bleb is often red at first, but the redness may disappear with time. You can see it by lifting the upper eyelid. You will also feel it if you touch it. However, there is nothing to worry about. The bleb is actually a reservoir of fluid that has drained from your eye. Its presence means your surgery was successful. The bleb may or may not disappear with time. It should be monitored regularly, and a few precautions are required to prevent infections that could have serious consequences, including loss of sight. Such infections develop mainly in cases of perforation of the bleb, as bacteria can enter easily when there is a leak in the bleb. Unfortunately, you will not be able to tell if you have such a leak. Ophthalmologists thus recommend that contact lenses not be worn if you have a filtering bleb, to reduce the risks of perforation. Regular check-ups, as recommended by your ophthalmologist, are crucial. In addition, you must go to emergency in case of pain, redness or pus in the eye, eyelids that stick together or deteriorated vision.

Trabecular bypass stent (iStent)

This new surgical option consists in installing an L-shaped implant approved by Health Canada in 2009. It is an increasingly popular option because it is minimally invasive.

The implant is 1 mm long and 0.33 mm wide. It is placed inside the canal of Schlemm through a small incision in the cornea. It lowers intraocular pressure by bypassing the trabecular meshwork and rerouting the aqueous humour from the anterior chamber directly into the canal of Schlemm (*Figure* ❻).

This procedure is frequently performed together with cataract surgery. This gives the best results, as cataract surgery slightly lowers intraocular pressure.

Suprachoroidal implant (gold micro shunt)

An implant in the suprachoroidal space (between the sclera and the choroid) can establish a connection between the anterior chamber and the suprachoroidal space.

The implant used for this surgery, the gold micro shunt, is a microplate of 24-carat gold containing nine channels. Once inserted and positioned, the gold micro shunt creates a new pathway for aqueous humour drainage above the choroid, where the humour is absorbed. The result is a drop in intraocular pressure. However, scarring may also occur after this type of surgery, and this can prevent the implant from working properly.

Cataract surgery (lens extraction)

This surgical procedure involves removing the lens and replacing it with an intraocular implant that takes up less space in the eye. This procedure is being increasingly used in angle-closure glaucoma. It creates space in the eye, so the iris no longer obstructs the trabecular meshwork, leading to better aqueous humour drainage.

In addition, it is not uncommon for patients with glaucoma to also have cataracts (clouding of the lens in the eye). For such patients, cataract surgery is required. The cataract surgery treats the glaucoma at the same time, as it generally lowers intraocular pressure by several mm Hg. However, as it does not generally

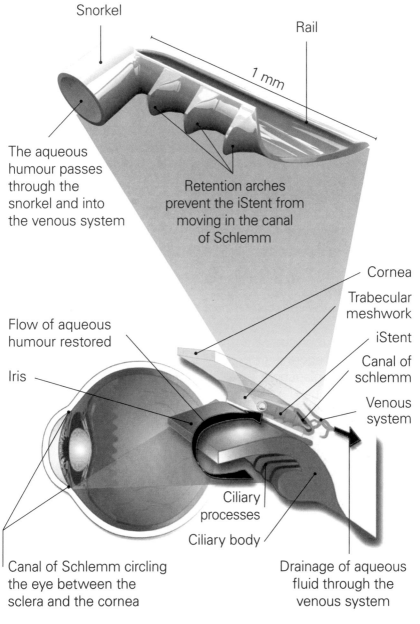

Snorkel

Rail

1 mm

The aqueous humour passes through the snorkel and into the venous system

Retention arches prevent the iStent from moving in the canal of Schlemm

Cornea

Trabecular meshwork

iStent

Flow of aqueous humour restored

Canal of schlemm

Iris

Venous system

Ciliary processes

Ciliary body

Canal of Schlemm circling the eye between the sclera and the cornea

Drainage of aqueous fluid through the venous system

❻ Trabecular bypass stent (iStent)

lower intraocular pressure enough to control glaucoma, another treatment (drops or surgery) may be required.

In some cases, however, the inflammation caused by the surgery and the post-operative use of cortisone can trigger a substantial increase in intraocular pressure, causing major damage—especially in advanced glaucoma. The ophthalmologist may then decide, if the patient agrees, to perform a combination surgery, that is, a non-penetrating deep sclerectomy (NPDS), a trabeculectomy, an ExPress Shunt, trabectome surgery, a trabecular stent bypass or laser cyclophotocoagulation at the same time as the cataract surgery.

Sometimes, a goniosynechialysis (the iris is pulled away from the trabecular meshwork, to which it is stuck) may also be performed at the same time as the cataract surgery in people with angle-closure glaucoma.

Vitrectomy

Vitrectomy is the surgical removal of the vitreous humour from the eye. The vitreous humour is not essential for vision and can be removed and replaced by a transparent liquid or, temporarily, by a gas. This procedure is performed in case of primary ciliary block angle-closure glaucoma (see *Chapter 2*) to prevent the vitreous humour from pushing the iris and the lens against the iridocorneal angle. Vitrectomy may also be performed when the vitreous humour has moved into the anterior chamber—as a result of trauma, for example.

How is surgery performed?

Surgical procedures to treat glaucoma are generally performed in a hospital under local anesthesia. They are not painful and last about 30 to 45 minutes. You may return home shortly after the surgery or you may have to spend a night in hospital. Immobilization for several hours or sometimes several days after the surgery may be required. There is a period of convalescence of one to two weeks during which you may not lift heavy loads or perform strenuous physical activities. It is also recommended that you avoid bending forward and stay out of swimming pools.

Your ophthalmologist will prescribe eye drops, which you must apply for several weeks to protect against infection and inflammation. It is also recommended that you wear something to protect your eyes at night (plastic eye shield, band over the eyes) temporarily.

Vision recovery after surgery is variable, and it can take several weeks.

Side effects of eye surgery

Complications during or after eye surgery are not common but they can be very severe. Before suggesting surgery, your ophthalmologist always looks at the risks involved. If your ophthalmologist suggests surgery, it is because he or she considers the risks of the disease to outweigh the possible adverse effects of the operation. What's more, there are solutions for dealing with most complications.

ONE PERSON'S STORY

Name: Michele	**Age:** 55 years old

Occupation: Massage Therapist

Five years ago, at age 50, Michele learned she had primary open-angle glaucoma. The ophthalmologist who made the diagnosis immediately prescribed prostaglandin analogue eye drops, to be applied in both eyes every evening at the same time to reduce her intraocular pressure, which was 32 mm Hg. Michele followed her doctor's instructions for two weeks. However, she quickly realized that the drops were causing her eyes to get red, the conjunctiva in particular, and she didn't like the way she looked. Besides, she hadn't noticed any change in her vision, as it had not been affected. She didn't see any reason to apply the drops every day because her vision was good. She quickly abandoned the treatment.

Four years later, however, Michele noticed that her vision had become blurry. She consulted her ophthalmologist once more. He found that her intraocular pressure was very elevated, at 39 mm Hg, and that her visual field had narrowed. The vision impairment was irreversible, and Michele had to stop driving. The doctor performed a selective laser trabeculoplasty to try to reduce her intraocular pressure, but the treatment did not lower the pressure sufficiently. Worried that her optical nerve might deteriorate, the ophthalmologist suggested a trabeculectomy.

Two months after the surgery, Michele's intraocular pressure returned to normal and stabilized at 12 mm Hg. As a result, she no longer has to apply drops in her eyes daily. She is being followed regularly by her ophthalmologist to make sure her intraocular pressure doesn't rise. She has found a job closer to her home, but she has to take public transit to get there, as her vision will never be completely restored.

CHAPTER 6

LIVING WITH GLAUCOMA

Though glaucoma is recognized as a leading cause of blindness in the world, most people who have the disease can lead a normal life if they are diagnosed early and follow treatment as prescribed. This means that if you have glaucoma, your quality of life will not differ much from that of someone without the disease, except if major damage to the optic nerve has progressed to the point of irreversible deterioration of vision. For advanced glaucoma and certain particular forms of glaucoma, however, there are certain guidelines you must follow.

PSYCHOLOGICAL IMPACT

Learning that you have glaucoma may give rise to a whole range of emotions—from worry to denial, loss of self-confidence and anger. The psychological impact of a diagnosis of glaucoma must not be ignored, and help from friends and family is sometimes necessary to accept the diagnosis and learn to live with the disease. It is important as well to feel free to ask your ophthalmologist questions and to learn about the disease. A good understanding of glaucoma makes it easier to live with it and to take good care of yourself. It also helps reduce the stress that may accompany the changes likely to occur over the course of the disease—when the ophthalmologist starts to consider surgery, for example.

Generally, the main changes in the lives of people with glaucoma are in connection with managing and monitoring the disease. For many, the only lifestyle changes after a diagnosis of glaucoma are having to see an ophthalmologist regularly and having to apply eye drops at the same time every day for life (see *How to put in your eye drops* in *Chapter 5*).

Depending on the stage and type of glaucoma, certain additional precautions may be required, as described later in this chapter.

It often takes some time after learning you have glaucoma to accept that you have the disease and thus be ready to accept treatment. However, once through this stage, it is crucial that you follow the treatment prescribed by your doctor. Many patients discontinue their treatment, mainly because they don't feel any symptoms and thus do not have the impression that the eye drops are doing anything for them. However, though the benefits may not be noticeable, the therapy is nonetheless essential to minimize the impact of the disease on your quality of life. It is thus extremely important not to discontinue prescribed treatment.

We are getting better and better at controlling glaucoma. New treatments are appearing regularly and these can stabilize intraocular pressure in people with glaucoma. However, patient motivation is crucial if stability is to be achieved. Following the recommendations of your ophthalmologist on a daily basis often means making lifestyle changes.

GETTING AROUND

Most people with glaucoma can get around easily. Mobility is a problem only in very rare cases where peripheral vision loss is substantial, that is, in advanced-stage glaucoma.

Driving a car

People in the early stages of glaucoma can keep their driver's licence for a very long time, as their vision is not affected.

Driving only becomes difficult and dangerous in very advanced glaucoma. If the damage to the optic nerve and the visual field loss are substantial, the ophthalmologist may decide that the patient is unable to drive safely and must give up his or her driver's licence permanently.

To retain the right to drive, the Canadian Ophthalmological Society recommends that private drivers have a visual field of no less than 120 degrees along the horizontal meridian with both eyes open and examined together. Standards vary, however, from one province to the next and are more stringent for commercial drivers, taxi drivers and emergency vehicle drivers. In Quebec, for example, visual acuity must be at least 6/15 (20/50) with both eyes open and examined together to be able to drive a road vehicle. In addition, Quebec's driver licensing bureau, the Société d'assurance automobile du Québec (SAAQ), automatically sends a form to drivers at age 75 (another at age 80 and subsequently every two years) that must be completed by an ophthalmologist or an optometrist. The SAAQ can refuse to grant a driver's licence if the visual field is too damaged.

Air travel

There is no danger in taking an airplane if you have glaucoma, nor are any special precautions required. Pressure is increased artificially on board aircraft to compensate for the natural drop in pressure at high altitudes.

On the other hand, if you are planning a trip that involves air travel very soon after surgery to treat glaucoma, it is best to speak to your ophthalmologist, even though air travel generally presents no risk.

SPORTS AND LEISURE

You can certainly practice sports if you have glaucoma. In fact, it is recommended, as physical activity causes intraocular pressure to drop slightly. Nonetheless, caution is required with certain sports. Sports that demand excessive exertion, for example, such as weight lifting, are contraindicated (not advised). Other types of sports are not formally contraindicated, except in pigmentary glaucoma. Vigorous exercise can cause more pigment to be released in people with this type of glaucoma, with the risk of blocking the trabecular meshwork and causing intraocular pressure to rise. However, an iridotomy (see *Chapter 5*) is an option that can make it possible for a person with pigmentary glaucoma to continue to engage in sports.

People who have had surgery for glaucoma (not including laser treatments) should avoid all sports activities in the month following the surgery as well as direct blows to the operated eye and contact with sea water or pool water.

Yoga

In yoga, it is mainly postures where the head is down and the feet up that are not advisable for people with glaucoma. Such postures can trigger a rise in intraocular pressure of 20 mm Hg, and holding the pose for several minutes could cause damage to the optic nerve.

Diving and downhill skiing

Diving in shallow water or in a pool does not significantly affect intraocular pressure, so such diving is not a problem.

Scuba diving is another matter. If you have glaucoma, you should consult your ophthalmologist first. Depending on the stage and type of glaucoma you have, your doctor can tell you if scuba diving might be dangerous for you. Deep-sea diving is to be avoided in advanced glaucoma, as the eyes may be subjected to considerable pressure during the descent. Scuba diving is also highly inadvisable in people who have just had surgery—a trabeculectomy or a deep sclerectomy (see *Chapter 5*), for example. Downhill skiing poses no risk for people with glaucoma.

Saunas
Saunas can be enjoyed without concern. Intraocular pressure tends to drop inside a sauna, but it returns to its original level within about an hour. However, there is no proof that saunas are beneficial for people with glaucoma.

Musical instruments
Like yoga, playing certain musical instruments can cause intraocular pressure to rise. The problem is mainly with wind instruments, such as a trumpet, which require a lot of breath and pressure. If you play such an instrument, or if you want to start playing one, you should consult your ophthalmologist.

LIFESTYLE AND NUTRITION

People with glaucoma can enjoy all the pleasures of life, like those who do not have it.

Diet
Though a diet rich in fruits and vegetables is always recommended to meet our bodies' need for vitamins and minerals, there is no particular diet that can reduce intraocular pressure for any length of time. It is not necessary, as a result, to take vitamin or nutritional supplements, as there is no proof that such supplements can prevent the onset or progression of glaucoma.

Coffee and tea

Coffee and tea have no effect on glaucoma when consumed in moderation. They can cause a slight increase in intraocular pressure in the first hour after consumption, but the increase is so minimal there is no reason to avoid drinking these beverages. The impact on intraocular pressure might be more significant, however, if you drank a large quantity of tea or coffee—or of any liquid, for that matter—in a very short time (say one litre in less than an hour). The recommendation is thus to drink smaller amounts over the course of the day.

Tobacco

The harmful health effects of smoking are well known. Smoking is the most significant risk factor in many diseases, cancer among

INTERACTIONS WITH OTHER DRUGS

If you have glaucoma, it is recommended that you read the notice that comes with any drug you are planning to take very carefully to make sure there is no risk for you. Or you can check with your ophthalmologist or your pharmacist.

Most medications can be taken without risk if you have open-angle glaucoma—except cortisone (oral, topical or spray), which can increase intraocular pressure. It is thus best to consult your ophthalmologist before taking cortisone.

If you are an angle-closure glaucoma suspect and you have not had an iridotomy, you must not take any drugs that cause pupil dilation, as this could result in an acute angle-closure glaucoma attack. Drugs that can cause pupil dilation include antidepressants, antipsychotics, certain cough suppressants, antispasmodics and antihistamines (anti-allergy medicines). If you have had an iridotomy, you can often use any of these medications without a problem. However, an iridotomy will not necessarily provide complete protection against an acute angle-closure glaucoma attack (see *Chapter 5*).

them. Though it has not been established beyond a doubt that tobacco is a risk factor in glaucoma, several recent studies show an association between glaucoma and smoking. It is thus preferable to not smoke.

Alcohol

If you have glaucoma, you can still enjoy alcohol, in moderation. Alcohol tends to lower not only intraocular pressure, but also blood pressure. However, alcohol cannot be considered "therapy" and it is not recommended that it be used as such given the possible undesirable side effects.

Cannabis

Like alcohol, cannabis (marijuana) tends to lower intraocular pressure. However, high doses must be consumed on a very frequent basis to obtain a beneficial effect on intraocular pressure. Studies to date on the medical use of cannabis to treat glaucoma demonstrate that it is less effective than treatments prescribed by ophthalmologists. The Canadian Ophthalmological Society does not support the medical use of marijuana for the treatment of glaucoma due to its short duration of action, the incidence of adverse effects and the absence of scientific evidence showing a beneficial effect on the course of the disease. Furthermore, cannabis also lowers blood pressure, and if blood pressure drops more than intraocular pressure, the optic nerve could be harmed.

GLAUCOMA AND OTHER EYE DISORDERS

It is not uncommon to have other eye diseases at the same time as glaucoma. At each check-up, your ophthalmologist will look for onset or progression of other eye diseases and may recommend surgery or treatment for such diseases that will not negatively affect your glaucoma.

Cataracts

Some people may develop cataracts in addition to glaucoma. In general, cataract surgery poses few risks for people with glaucoma. In fact, the ophthalmologist/surgeon may opt for combination surgery for the cataract and the glaucoma to restore the best possible vision and reduce intraocular pressure at the same time. If the ophthalmologist/surgeon decides to operate on the cataract only, the surgery may nonetheless lower intraocular pressure by about 2 mm Hg.

Age-related macular degeneration (AMD)

Glaucoma and AMD are diseases whose onset is generally after age 40. In other words, it is not uncommon to have both as we age. This combination of diseases, however, can be very disabling, as AMD affects central vision and glaucoma affects peripheral vision. Fortunately, there are medications for both diseases that do not interfere with one another.

Dry eyes

With age, our eyes tend to become drier. It's not so much the amount of tears we produce as their quality, because those we produce when we are older do not protect the cornea as well as those we produced when we were younger. People complain that their eyes tear, itch and burn. In such cases, artificial tears should be applied several times a day. Artificial tears are not a problem if you have glaucoma, even if you already use eye drops to control intraocular pressure. However, artificial tears without BAK (an antibacterial agent already present in certain eye drops used to treat glaucoma) may be recommended. BAK toxicity can develop in the eye when too many drops with BAK are applied.

LOW VISION REHABILITATION

The risk of going blind due to glaucoma is very small, especially if your disease is detected early and you carefully follow the treatment prescribed. However, advanced glaucoma can affect your visual field by altering your side or peripheral vision, though you will continue to see what is in front of you (central vision is retained for a long time). Because of the reduced visual field, you could end up bumping into things and having difficulty driving and walking down stairs.

Low vision rehabilitation with the help of a vision rehabilitation specialist cannot restore lost eyesight if your glaucoma is in a very advanced stage. Such a specialist can, however, help you with visual strategies that will allow you to make the most of your remaining vision. Low vision rehabilitation involves training in the use of vision aids such as magnifiers, telescopes, special lights, filters, adapted television stations, special software, touch pads, e-book readers, audio books, big button telephones, etc. And if you are still

CONTACT LENSES

Intraocular pressure is not affected by wearing contact lenses. This means that wearing contact lenses is not a problem if you have glaucoma unless you have had filtration surgery for open-angle glaucoma (trabeculectomy or deep sclerectomy). These procedures create a filtering bleb, a little bubble or bulge that appears under the upper eyelid (see *Chapter 5*). If you have a bleb, it is unadvisable to wear contact lenses, as the edges of most lenses can pierce a bleb and cause complications.

Soft contact lenses tend to absorb drops applied to the eyes to treat glaucoma. This can cause adverse effects (dryness or irritation of the eye, or even deterioration of the contact lens). It is thus recommended that contact lenses be removed before applying eye drops and put back 15 to 20 minutes later.

Interactions with certain eye drops are also a possibility. As a result, you must ask your ophthalmologist if there are any precautions you need to take.

working, a low vision rehabilitation specialist can also help you arrange a redesign of your work station or an occupation reclassification by your employer. An orientation and mobility (O&M) specialist can also teach you orientation and mobility exercises that will help you get around more easily.

In Canada, vision rehabilitation services are offered free of charge in specialized centres based on certain criteria (field of vision affected, visual acuity, etc.).

TELEVISION AND COMPUTER SCREENS

Watching television or spending time in front of a computer cannot cause or aggravate glaucoma. However, if your vision is impaired you may have difficulty focusing on a screen for long periods of time or reading small characters. Fortunately, there is software available to help you read or write documents on a computer.

Screen magnifiers
These programs magnify text, graphics and images displayed on a computer screen and let you adjust the degree of magnification.

Screen readers
These programs convert printed documents (books, newspaper articles, etc.) that have been scanned into electronic documents that can be saved on a computer. The programs can even read electronic documents out loud, magnify the text on screen and modify the colour contrast to improve visibility.

PREGNANCY AND BREASTFEEDING
Women being treated for glaucoma must tell their ophthalmologist as soon as possible if they become pregnant or are planning to become pregnant. The ophthalmologist may decide to discontinue or modify the treatment.

There are still many questions about treatments to use for glaucoma in women who are pregnant or nursing. Fortunately, however, intraocular pressure tends to decrease during pregnancy and certain medications can be stopped.

To date, there are no studies demonstrating the effects on a human fetus of the medications used to treat primary or secondary open-angle glaucoma, but carbonic anhydrase inhibitors have caused malformation in mice. Prostaglandin analogues may also increase the risk of premature delivery and are thus often stopped after the second trimester. Trabeculoplasty may be a good drug-free alternative.

On the other hand, if there is major damage to the optic nerve, or if intraocular pressure is very elevated, it may be advisable to continue treatment. The ophthalmologist will select the treatment he or she feels is best under the circumstances, generally opting for medications with which he or she has considerable experience. Certain measures can also be taken to reduce absorption of the drug into the general circulation (see box *What if I am pregnant or breastfeeding?* in *Chapter 5*).

Breastfeeding mothers must understand that drugs they take pass into their breast milk. The ophthalmologist will select a treatment together with the patient or decide to discontinue all treatment. As with pregnancy, the ophthalmologist weighs the benefits and risks of glaucoma treatment.

CHAPTER 7
TREATMENTS
OF THE FUTURE

Glaucoma research is very active at present and is in constant need of grants and donations. Advances are being made rapidly, giving hope that future treatments will be even more effective in limiting complications and repairing lesions caused by glaucoma and that one day it might be possible to prevent onset of the disease. With the extraordinary progress in research on new therapies, no one can predict today how glaucoma will be treated in ten or even five years. Now more than ever, the future looks promising, not only for early diagnosis and treatment of glaucoma but also for repair of eyes damaged by the disease.

FUTURE DRUGS

Though they are effective in lowering intraocular pressure, the medications currently available often have adverse effects, such as dry, red or inflamed eyes. Scientists are working to identify new substances that will make it possible for pharmaceutical companies to offer eye drops that are better tolerated, applied less frequently or delivered in different ways (for example, in drug-eluting contact lenses, punctal plugs or long-lasting injections).

Other drugs are also being studied that might be effective in repairing damage to the optic nerve caused by the glaucoma. A number of research teams are working on drugs that could protect nerves associated with vision (drugs with neuroprotective potential) so that medications to preserve or repair the optic nerve can be developed.

PERSONALIZED MEDICINE

Personalized medicine is a new approach that calls for selecting treatment based on the patient's genetic profile. With a genetic profile, treatment can be more targeted, safer and more effective. The goal? The right treatment, for the right patient, at the right time.

As we do not yet know the exact cause of the elevated intraocular pressure characteristic of glaucoma, researchers the world over are trying to determine the genes involved in the disease. Discovery of one or more genes responsible for glaucoma will make it possible to develop new treatments adapted to patient genetic profiles. It will also make early identification of those at risk possible.

DIAGNOSTIC IMAGING AND SURGICAL TECHNIQUES

Many studies are being conducted to develop new imaging technologies that can improve glaucoma diagnosis. In particular, researchers are looking at ways to identify the exact location of the blockage in the drainage system in the eyes of people with glaucoma. Researchers are also busy developing new microinvasive surgical techniques (canal of Schlemm stenting, for example) that will make it possible to treat glaucoma earlier, before scarring or atrophy of eye tissue occurs.

NEW IMPLANTS

A number of drug-delivery implants are currently under development to improve the treatment of glaucoma, sustained-release intraocular implants in particular. Placed inside the eye, these implants would make it possible to release over months a drug that acts on intraocular pressure. Such implants would replace the eye drops that have to be applied daily and would mean better treatment compliance.

Other types of implants are also being studied, in particular an implant that would allow the ophthalmologist to control and adjust intraocular pressure. This implant is equipped with a tube through which the aqueous humour can drain, and its opening is controlled by a metal disk. By adjusting the opening, the ophthalmologist can allow more or less aqueous humour to drain depending on intraocular pressure measurements.

GENE THERAPY

Gene therapy alters the genetic material of cells involved in disease. The structure of the defective gene in the cell is modified to prevent onset of the disease or make cells more resistant to it.

A viral vector is used to introduce a suitable genetic code. The virus must have the ability to penetrate the cell and insert its DNA in host chromosomes. The patient's cells can then produce the proteins that fight or correct glaucoma.

The challenge is to prevent disease progression by targeting the molecules involved.

Gene therapy is a future treatment for prevention of glaucoma, but additional studies are required to develop clinical applications. Though still in the experimental stage, gene therapies may nonetheless become available for people with glaucoma in the not so distant future.

STEM CELL TRANSPLANTATION

Nerve cell transplants are not a feasible option at present for people with glaucoma. However, scientists hope to be able one day to repair damage to the optic nerve caused by glaucoma by producing cells from blood and bone marrow samples taken from the patient and then transplanting them in the eyes. Some researchers thus believe stem cell transplantation may be able to restore vision in people with glaucoma, even in the advanced stage.

Transplantation of stem cells genetically modified to produce genes that protect against glaucoma or its progression is another possibility.

These procedures involve long-term research. We do not expect to be transplanting stem cells in the near future, as there are still technical problems. Nonetheless there is reason for much hope.

USEFUL ADDRESSES

CANADA

Accessible Media Inc. (AMI)
1-800-567-6755
www.ami.ca

AMI is a multimedia organization operating two broadcast services, AMI-audio and AMI-tv, and a multi-functional website for the purpose of bringing media in an alternate form to those not able to follow in traditional ways.

Canadian Association of Optometrists (CAO)
234 Argyle Avenue
Ottawa, ON K2P 1B9
1-613-235-7924 or 1-888-263-4676
www.opto.ca

Professional association of optometrists in Canada. It is also the national federation of 10 provincial associations of optometrists.

Canadian Ophthalmological Society

610-1525 Carling Avenue
Ottawa, ON K1Z 8R9
1-800-267-5763
www.eyesite.ca

Canadian association of physicians and surgeons specializing in eye care.

CNIB

1929 Bayview Avenue
Toronto, ON M4G 3E8
1-800-563-2642
www.cnib.ca

Nationwide, community-based, registered charity committed to research, public education and vision health for all Canadians. CNIB Library offers access to thousands of titles in Braille and PrintBraille as well as audio books, newspapers and magazine, descriptive videos and document search services. Alternate-media books and other documents can be consulted online or delivered on loan postage-free.

Glaucoma Research Society of Canada

1929 Bayview Avenue, Suite 215E
Toronto, ON M4G 3E8
1-416-483-0200 or 1-877-483-0204
www.glaucomaresearch.ca

National registered charity dedicated to funding glaucoma research. Website provides information about glaucoma.

QUEBEC

Association des établissements de réadaptation en déficience physique du Québec (AERDPQ)
1001, boulevard De Maisonneuve Ouest, bureau 430
Montréal (QC) H3A 3C8
1-514-282-4205
www.aerdpq.org

Association of centres in the province of Quebec for rehabilitation of physical disabilities offering specialized rehabilitation services, for people with vision impairments in particular. Here is a list of centres by region.

Centre de protection et de réadaptation de la Côte-Nord
835, boulevard Jolliet
Baie-Comeau (QC) G5C 1P5
1-418-589-9927 or 1-866-389-2038
www.cprcn.qc.ca

Centre de réadaptation de la Gaspésie
230, route du Parc
Sainte-Anne-des-Monts (QC) G4V 2C4
1-418-763-3325 or 1-855-763-3325
www.crgaspesie.qc.ca

Centre de réadaptation en déficience physique Chaudière-Appalaches
9500, boulevard du Centre-Hospitalier
Charny (QC) G6X 0A1
1-418-380-2064
TDD: 1-418-380-2089
www.crdpca.qc.ca

Centre de réadaptation en déficience physique Le Bouclier
1075, boulevard Firestone, bureau 1000
Joliette (QC) J6E 6X6
1-450-755-2741 or 1-800-363-2783
TDD: 1-450-759-8763
www.bouclier.qc.ca

Centre de réadaptation en déficience physique Le Parcours
2230, rue de l'Hôpital – C.P. 1200
Jonquière (QC) G7X 7X2
1-418-695-7700
www.csssjonquiere.qc.ca

Centre de réadaptation Estrie
300, rue King Est, bureau 200
Sherbrooke (QC) J1G 1B1
1-819-346-8411
TTY: 1-819-821-0247
www.centredereadaptationestrie.org

Centre de réadaptation InterVal
1775, rue Nicolas-Perrot
Trois-Rivières (QC) G9A 1C5
1-819-378-4083
www.centreinterval.qc.ca

Centre de réadaptation La Maison
100, chemin Docteur-Lemay
Rouyn-Noranda (QC) J9X 5T2
1-819-762-6592
www.crlm.qc.ca

Centre de réadaptation MAB-Mackay
7000, rue Sherbrooke Ouest
Montréal (QC) H4B 1R3
1-514-488-5552
www.mabmackay.ca

Centre régional de réadaptation La RessourSe
135, boulevard Saint-Raymond
Gatineau (QC) J8Y 6X7
1-819-777-3293
TTY: 1-819-777-5465
www.crr-la-ressourse.qc.ca

Centre régional de réadaptation L'interAction
800, avenue du Sanatorium
Mont-Joli (QC) G5H 3L6
1-418-775-7261 or 1-855-605-3235
www.csssmitis.ca/interaction

Institut de réadaptation en déficience physique de Québec (IRDPQ)
525, boulevard Wilfrid-Hamel
Québec (QC) G1M 2S8
1-418-529-9141
TDD/TTY: 1-418-649-3733
www.irdpq.qc.ca

Institut Nazareth & Louis-Braille
1111, rue Saint-Charles Ouest – Tour Ouest, 2e étage
Longueuil (QC) J4K 5G4
1-450-463-1710 or 1-800-361-7063
www.inlb.qc.ca

Association des médecins ophtalmologistes du Québec (AMOQ)

2, Complexe Desjardins – C.P. 216, succursale Desjardins
Montréal (QC) H5B 1G8
1-514-350-5124
www.amoq.org

Quebec association of ophthalmologists. The Web site provides information for the public.

Association des optométristes du Québec (AOQ)

1265, rue Berri, bureau 740
Montréal (QC) H2L 4X4
1-514-288-6272 or 1-888-SOS-OPTO (1-888-767-6786)
www.aoqnet.qc.ca

Quebec association of optometrists. The Web site provides information for the public.

Audiothèque

4765, 1re Avenue, bureau 210
Québec (QC) G1H 2T3
1-418-627-8882 or 1-877-393-0103
Montreal region: 1-514-393-0103
www.audiotheque.com

Information centre for people who cannot access written materials. Offers telephone access to readings of newspaper articles, magazines, circulars and other written material.

Centre de réadaptation, d'orientation et d'intégration au travail (AIM CROIT)
750, boulevard Marcel-Laurin, bureau 450
Saint-Laurent (QC) H4M 2M4
1-514-744-2944
TDD: 1-514-744-2613
www.aimcroitqc.org

Accommodated job search assistance for people with visual impairments and workplace adaptation assistance for employers.

CNIB
3044, rue Delisle
Montréal (QC) H4C 1M9
1-514-934-4622 or 1-800-465-4622
Quebec region: 1-418-204-1124
www.inca.ca

Nationwide, community-based, registered charity committed to research, public education and vision health for all Canadians.

Comité d'adaptation de la main-d'œuvre (CAMO)
55, avenue du Mont-Royal Ouest
Bureau 300, 3e étage
Montréal (QC) H2T 2S6
1-514-522-3310 or 1-888-522-3310
TDD: 1-514-522-5425
www.camo.qc.ca

Provincial committee whose mission is to promote access to training and employment for people living with disabilities.

Institut de réadaptation en déficience physique de Québec (IRDPQ)

525, boulevard Wilfrid-Hamel
Québec (QC) G1M 2S8
1-418-529-9141
TDD/TTY: 1-418-649-3733
www.irdpq.qc.ca

Offers a rehabilitation program for people with visual impairments and access to optical aids to compensate for visual loss.

Institut Nazareth & Louis-Braille (INLB)

1111, rue Saint-Charles Ouest – Tour Ouest, 2e étage
Longueuil (QC) J4K 5G4
1-450-463-1710 or 1-800-361-7063
Consult the Web site for service points in Montreal, Laval and Saint-Jean-sur-Richelieu.
www.inlb.qc.ca

Specializes in low vision rehabilitation. Member of the Association des établissements de réadaptation en déficience physique du Québec (AERDPQ). Offers services for people with total or partial vision loss.

The Quebec Glaucoma Foundation

4135, rue de Rouen
Montréal (QC) H1V 1G5
514-259-4229
www.fondationglaucomequebec.com

Promotes glaucoma research in Quebec and provides information for people with glaucoma.

Service québécois du livre adapté (SQLA)
475, boulevard De Maisonneuve Est
Montréal (QC) H2L 5C4
1-514-873-4454 or 1-866-410-0844
www.banq.qc.ca/sqla/index.html

A French-language adapted book collection (Braille and audio books) available at the Grande Bibliothèque.

Vues & Voies (formerly La Magnétothèque)
1055, boulevard René-Lévesque Est, bureau 501
Montréal (QC) H2L 4S5
1-514-282-1999 or 1-800-361-0635
www.vuesetvoix.com

Close to 10,000 audio books: novels, philosophy, psychology, biographies, etc. Volunteers also read editorials and articles from Quebec newspapers.

UNITED STATES

American Glaucoma Society
P.O. Box 193940
San Francisco, CA 94119
1-415-561-8587
www.americanglaucomasociety.net

Children's Glaucoma Foundation
Two Longfellow Place, Suite 201
Boston, Massachusetts 02114
1-617-227-3011
www.childrensglaucoma.com

The Glaucoma Foundation
80 Maiden Lane, Suite 700
New York, NY 10038
1-212-285-0080
www.glaucomafoundation.org

Glaucoma Research Foundation
251 Post Street, Suite 600
San Francisco, CA 94108
1-415-986-3162 or 1-800-826-6693
www.glaucoma.org

WEB SITES

www.audible.com (in English)
www.audible.fr (in French)

Sites for digital download of audiobooks for playback on telephones, mp3-players, tablets and other devices.